Essenti

Beg

100+ Essential Oil Recipes And How To Use The Essential Oils To Maximise Your Health And Longevity

By Amy Joyson

are for clarifying purposes only and are the owned by the owners themselves, not affiliated with this document.

Disclaimer – Please read!
The information provided in this book is designed to provide helpful information on the subjects discussed. This book is not meant to be used, nor should it be used, to diagnose or treat any medical condition. For diagnosis or treatment of any medical problem, consult your own physician. The publisher and author are not responsible for any specific health or allergy needs that may require medical supervision and are not liable for any damages or negative consequences from any treatment, action, application or preparation, to any person reading or following the information in this book. References are provided for informational purposes only and do not constitute endorsement of any websites or other sources. Readers should be aware that the websites listed in this book may change.

Table of Contents

Chapter 5 – Advanced massage treatments for applying Essential Oils

Essential Oils Recipes For Your Pets 195

Introduction

The essential oils can be quite a daunting prospect when first looking into them. There is after all over 90 of them! This eBook is the perfect introduction to the world of essential oils. From answering basic questions and providing background on the art of aromatherapy, to detailed remedies and recipes for solving common health issues. This guide contains everything you need to know to unlock the incredible healing power of these natural products.

Importantly, there is no 'presumed knowledge' expected of the reader; that is, even if you know *absolutely nothing* about essential oils, you won't be overwhelmed by technical terms or jargon. However, you can also expect that once you reach the end of this book, you will feel confident enough to begin improving the health of yourself and others with the power of essential oils.

The potential health benefits that can be gained through proper use of the oils is outstanding. Bergamot Oil is often used to increase alertness, while the essential oils of Lavender and Geranium are used to promote restfulness. There are oils that can be used as an anti-depressant and other oils that can be used to cure the common cold. The applications are almost endless and I hope you find that you are opened up to this world by the end of the book.

Thanks for choosing this book, I truly hope you both learn from and enjoy it!

Chapter 1 – What are Essential Oils?

History of essential oils

For thousands of years, essential oils have been used in various cultures to cure ailments and alleviate symptoms associated with illness. The Ancient Egyptians were perhaps one of the first great civilizations to regularly use essential oils for their therapeutic effects, amongst other varied applications (such as food preparation, beauty treatments and religious ceremonies). For example, some essential oils, such as myrrh, were used for their anti-bacterial properties and were an important part of the embalming process. This practice of using essential oils for their therapeutic properties passed from the Egyptians to the Greeks, who used them extensively in massage and aromatherapy. Essential oils even won the endorsement of famed Greek physician Hippocrates, commonly known as the 'father of medicine'. He was among those who prescribed their therapeutic use in these areas as part of a holistic approach to patient health. Later, the Romans also began to utilize the power of essential oils for therapeutic purposes, using them in the purification of religious and political buildings, and in steam baths as a prophylactic against disease. Essential oils had such high value in ancient times that they are claimed to be two of the three remarkable items (frankincense and myrrh) gifted at the birth of Jesus by the Three Wise Men. Indeed, essential oils were important and valuable trade commodities for many nations.

During the Dark and Middle Ages, mystics commonly used the healing power of essential oils to treat medical complaints, although their therapeutic use was largely relegated to the fringes of medicine at this time. It was not until the modern era that essential oils enjoyed a renaissance of sorts, with their championing by French chemist René Gattefossé during the early part of the 20th century. (He was, in fact, the man to first coin the term 'aromatherapy' – the practice by which essential oils and other aromatic substances are administered for therapeutic purposes). Parisian doctor, Jean Valnet, also used essential oils therapeutically to treat patients during WWII. His work in this area was connected to research by two of his contemporaries, Dr. Jean-Claude Lapraz and Dr. Paul Belaiche, who determined through research that the healing properties of essential oils were thanks to their antibacterial, antiviral, antiseptic and antifungal qualities. More recent studies have further confirmed these findings. Today, the use of essential oils for their therapeutic effects has gained a significant following, and the practice of aromatherapy is subscribed to by millions. In an age of advanced and industrialized medicine, many are returning to ancient natural methods to seek a way to best maintain, repair and improve our physical selves.

What are essential oils?

Simply put, essential oils are the concentrated essences (hence, the use of the term 'essential') of aromatic compounds. In Ancient China, these plant and flower essences were believed to constitute the 'soul' of the organism. These are often clear liquids and, contrary to the 'oil' in their name, often have a consistency more like that of water than of typical oils. From herbs, to flowers, to fruits, essential oils can be derived from many different organic sources. Around 400-500 essential oils are produced commercially, although there are many more types available. Essential oils are typically very complex, with single varieties often containing hundreds of individual aromatic compounds. As essential oils are derived from natural sources, they contain no harmful or synthetic chemicals which can have unknown detrimental effects on the body.

Essential oils are a key ingredient in many of today's consumer products, particularly in foodstuffs and cosmetics. They are also the subject around which the practice of aromatherapy is based. Essential oils hold great appeal to the individual due to their accessibility and usefulness. Not only can they be applied therapeutically, but also in foods, for household cleaning solutions, or simply for their distinctive aromatic properties. There are few tinctures which have such numerous practical applications, and are locked within the natural world that surrounds us, ready to be released.

How are essential oils obtained?

The process of extracting essential oils varies, largely depending upon the source material and available technologies. The oldest and perhaps simplest method of extracting essential oils is a process known as *enfleurage*. A relatively simple method, this involves crushing the product from which the oils are to be derived, and mixing the resulting powder or paste with a lipid (such as olive or vegetable oil). The oils from the source product permeate the lipids, and the essential oil infused mixture is then processed to be separated from the product residue. Though yielding a rather crude final result, this was a common method due to the lack of knowledge and expertise surrounding more complex extractions. The process for exploiting essential oils became more sophisticated over time. Archaeological evidence from the Middle East, such as pottery stills containing the residue of aromatic compounds, indicates that advanced extraction techniques were already being practiced in ancient times. Today, more sophisticated extraction methods mean that we can obtain highly pure and refined essential oils. The most pure essential oils are obtained through a process of steam distillation, whereby a solution is made from the source product, which is then heated, evaporating the essential oils. These are later collected through condensation after being cooled further along the system. The purity of essential oils is especially important when it comes to their therapeutic administration.

Another technique used for obtaining essential oils is the use of *solvents*. The use of chemical solvents is generally unfavorable amongst professional aromatherapists as it is the least natural way of extracting essential oils. The idea behind the method is that all the solvents used in the extraction are removed but occasionally light chemical traces will be left in the product. In this method the plant from which the essential oil is to be sourced is dissolved in a chemical solvent. The most common solvents used are; methylene chloride, hexane and benzene. These solvents have a lower boiling point than the essential oils and so are evaporated off, leaving behind the pure essential oil.

One of the most popular methods of obtaining essential oils is *steam distillation*. It is a simple procedure in which freshly harvested plants are suspended above a vat of boiling water. The steam that emerges from the water extracts the oil from the plant. The rising steam is captured and pushed through a tube before being cooled. As the steam condenses back into water, the essential oil (which doesn't mix with water) separates away.

Obtaining 'therapeutic grade' essential oils

In order to enjoy the therapeutic benefit of essential oils, it is vital that a product that is both high in purity and quality is used. However, essential oils that meet these requirements can be very expensive, due to the fact that a very high amount of organic matter is required to produce each milliliter of oil. In addition to this, it is much cheaper to extract the oils when sub-standard techniques are used. Typically, the extraction technique that results in the best quality oils requires both expensive distillation equipment and the expertise of a professional trained in its operation to perform the extraction. Sadly, the market for essential oils is severely lacking in regulation. Although, on the one hand this means that essential oils are readily obtainable, on the other, it makes certification of the quality of the product for sale difficult to verify for the individual. Therefore, as consumers of these important commodities, there are certain things we should look for, especially when shopping online for essential oils for therapeutic use:

- Is the information relating to the product thoroughly and adequately provided? E.g. Is the Latin name of the plant genus provided? Is the source of origin of the extract given?

- Does the product information state that the oils are 100% pure? Is there a suggestion that oils have been adulterated with other substances?

- When you receive the product, is it adequately and correctly labelled? Does the product smell as you would expect it to smell?

- Is the product significantly cheaper than normal market prices? If so, it is likely that the quality or purity of the product is compromised. (If it seems too good to be true, it usually is)

- Does the vendor seem legitimate? Do they appear to be knowledgeable about the product they are selling? Does the vendor seem trustworthy?

- Is the vendor you are purchasing the product from well-reviewed? If possible, try to find review of the company by third parties rather than relying on those that appear on their own website.

Although it can be difficult to guarantee that we are buying a legitimate product, particularly when shopping online, this can be true of any item – not just essential oils. It is important to carry out these basic precautions to protect ourselves as consumers, and to ensure that we are using a product of the highest quality. Remember; if you have reasons to suspect that the quality of an essential oil you have purchased is compromised *do not administer it therapeutically!*

How much should I be paying for essential oils?

As alluded to above, the comparative price of an essential oil is almost always reflective of its quality. However, there is no 'set price' for essential oils as such. All differ based on the expensiveness of the source material from which they are derived, and the volume of material required to produce one milliliter of essential oil. For example, take the case of essence of lemon. A large number of lemons are indeed required to produce one standard bottle of essence of lemon; however, because lemons are relatively inexpensive, it is normally one of the cheaper essential oils. A suggestion would be to compare the price of the oil you are looking to purchase to other reputable sites on the internet to make sure the price is in line.

How are essential oils administered?

Essential oils can be administered in a number of different ways. One of the most basic and effective methods (depending on the symptom being treated) is through topical application. This is not only true for treating topical conditions (e.g. such as skin irritation or bruising) but is also often a way to treat internal complaints (e.g. such as headaches or nausea). This method is connected to perhaps one of the most traditional ways to deliver therapeutic treatment in conjunction with massage therapy. When applied to the skin, essential oils are absorbed relatively quickly, as they are made up of very small molecules that are easily drawn into the dermis. This means that they are able to enter the bloodstream and take effect very quickly, compared to other therapeutic treatments.

A second way to administer essential oils is via either direct or indirect inhalation. In the case of the former, a personal inhaler is loaded with the oil(s) and their vapor is inhaled through the nose or mouth. For the latter, a vaporizer is typically employed, where the vapor of the oil(s) is diffused throughout a room. These methods are often best when treating an issue related to respiratory function, colds or flus, or sinus complaints. The final and perhaps least common method of administering essential oils is via ingestion. Though this technique can be suitable to obtain specific therapeutic results, it can be less safe than the above methods, particularly when not practiced or prescribed by a trained professional. Certain essential oils can damage the liver or kidneys when taken internally, or can interact with certain medications. Additionally, contraindications can occur when essential oils are processed through the digestive system. Always seek the advice of a trained professional if planning to administer essential oils via this method.

How do essential oils work?

From the three main ways that essential oils enter the body (dermally, or through inhalation or ingestion), the active ingredients interact with the body's systems in different ways. When taken through the skin, or via ingestion, the compounds from essential oils enter the blood stream acting much like a regular drug. They then circulate throughout the body and can have a localized effect on symptoms. Also when ingested, the ingredients from the oils are processed through the digestive system before being circulated through blood to the rest of the body.

When inhaled through the nose or mouth, essential oils interact with a number of different systems in the body. The olfactory system is responsible for controlling and effecting the sense of smell. As essential oils are highly aromatic, their interaction with the olfactory system can be an important part of their therapeutic application. Inhaled molecules also interact directly with the respiratory system, which can be a useful method of delivery when treating complaints associated with the respiratory tract and the lungs.

Finally, inhaled oils are believed to achieve some of their therapeutic outcomes by interacting with various receptors in the brain which constitute the limbic system. This system is thought to be responsible for a range of physiological responses, including heart rate, blood pressure, memory, breathing, and stress and hormone levels. This helps to explain why essential oils can have a profound array of effects on both human physiology and emotional well-being.

Why aren't essential oils backed as 'therapeutic drugs' by federal regulators?

One of the main issues surrounding universal acceptance of the 'therapeutic drug' status of essential oils relates to the dearth of clinical research evidence associated with them. However, this is not due to a lack of a link between essential oils and quantifiable therapeutic effect, but is primarily related to the fact that the number of clinical studies actually conducted in the area of essential oils has been limited. Many advocates of the therapeutic properties of essential oils claim that this is a result of two key factors. The first is due to the fact that drug companies have limited interest in sponsoring clinical trials in this area, due to a limited potential for profit. There is little to no money to be made from essential oils within the pharmaceutical industry, as they are natural products derived from natural sources, and therefore, are not patentable. Patents on drug design and manufacture are the number one source of revenue in the pharmaceutical industry.

Relatedly, the process for having drugs tested and certified by federal drug regulators is typically prohibitively expensive and depends upon the backing of the multibillion dollar pharmaceutical industry in some form. Thus, because backing by federal drug regulators *and* the pharmaceutical industry (who, because of the above may see the widespread therapeutic use of essential oils as contrary to their financial interests) are requisite for mainstream acceptance of therapeutic treatments, essential oils face a legitimacy problem. However, thanks to the limited clinical studies which *have* been conducted into essential oils thus far, we know that many of these products do in fact have clear antibacterial, antiviral and antifungal properties. This means that they can have a quantifiable effect on treating certain illnesses and conditions. Additionally, studies conducted on laboratory animals have shown that exposure to certain aromas under stressful conditions can improve behavioral and immune response. Finally, the amount of anecdotal evidence surrounding the positive therapeutic effects of essential oils is enormous. While not certifiable (as in the case of clinical evidence), this widespread popular backing nonetheless suggests that a significant multitude of people have used essential oils with great therapeutic results.

Essential oils and safety

It is important to know how to use essential oils correctly as their improper use can be harmful to your health. The following points should always be taken into consideration whenever using essential oils:

- Due to the fact that essential oils contain highly concentrated chemical compounds, they can cause irritation to the skin.

- Exposure to very high levels of concentrated essential oils (as with most very pure chemical compounds) can be toxic (if ingested), and may lead to damage of the liver and other organs.

- It is extremely important to practice using essential oils correctly and (normally) in diluted concentrations.

- Some essential oils may induce photosensitivity or be phototoxic. This increases your chances of experiencing sunburn or skin irritation during sun exposure after these oils have been applied. If you are unsure whether a particular essential oil may lead to such symptoms, you should avoid sun exposure after use.

- When essential oils are used with children, they should be diluted *below* the recommended dosage for adults. Although there are exceptions for some essential oils, it is best to avoid using with children until at least six years old. Essential oils should be stored safely and kept out of reach of children, and should only be administered to children by adults educated in their use.

- People with allergies should test diluted essential oils on a small area of skin before they are used topically. Wait one hour and if there are no symptoms of adverse reaction, you may proceed with therapeutic treatment.

- Essential oils should be kept away from the face, especially the eyes and ears. Essential oils will generally absorb into the skin after half an hour, so contact with these and other sensitive areas should be avoided immediately after use.

- Pregnant and breastfeeding women should avoid using essential oils.

- Sufferers of asthma should avoid administering essential oils via inhalation.

- Always consult your physician before beginning any treatment involving essential oils.

Despite all of these recommended precautions, clinical safety studies have shown there are very few bad side effects associated with the therapeutic use of essential oils, when used as directed. The fact that many essential oils are used pervasively in many commercial (and regulation approved) industries indicates their general level of safety.

Chapter 2 – The 30 Most Popular Essential Oils

As mentioned earlier, the amount of essential oils available with therapeutic applications number in the hundreds, and can be obtained from a vast array of organic matter. Many have overlapping properties, while others are distinct in their unique therapeutic potential. The following is a detailed list of the 30 most popular of these, including some common uses for each.

Lavender (Lavandula Angustifolia.)

Grown mainly for the extraction and use of its essential oil, lavender (*Lavandula*) has distinctive purple flowers and silver/green foliage. Seen as one of the most versatile essential oils, lavender has a long history of widespread therapeutic usage because of its various potential applications. For example, it is often used for its relaxing and calming properties; inversely, it can be a source of energy and invigoration. French scientist – sometimes referred to as the 'father of aromatherapy' - René Gattefossé famously identified lavender's potential for use as a treatment for irritated skin after he suffered severe burns in a laboratory explosion. This is due to lavender's properties as an anti-bacterial and anti-inflammatory agent, and can also be used as a treatment for minor cuts and bruises as a result. It is one of the few essential oils that can be used neat in some instances – however you should only do so after consulting a trained professional. Lavender is truly an *essential* essential oil, and one that no home should be without.

Lavender use has been recorded for over 2,500 years. Phoenicians, Egyptians and the people of Arabia would use lavender for mummification and perfume. Lavender was even used to cure a wide array of ailments (from back aches to insomnia) in ancient Greece.

As time passed, lavender became a prized commodity, and in ancient Roman times a pound of lavender flowers were sold for a month's wage of a farm laborer. The Romans used the lavender to scent their bath water, as well as an insect repellent, flavoring and perfume. The dried lavender was added to their smoking mixtures. In Renaissance and Medieval Europe, they covered the castles' stone floors with lavender. This would not only deodorize the floor, but it would also act as a disinfectant. Lavender was even grown in the infirmarian's garden, with the intended purpose of warding off diseases. During the Great Plague of London, which occurred in the 17th century, people would attach lavender bunches to their wrists to keep the Black Death at bay.

Lavandula angustifolia is the official name for English lavender (which most people think of as true lavender), while Lavendin is a hybrid between English and Spike Lavender. English lavender has little to no camphor in it. Spike Lavender, however, has about 40-percent camphor in it. And the hybrid of English and Spike lavender has about 20-percent camphor in it. Camphor is not a mild soothing agent, can be irritating on burns and some people are even allergic to it. That is why you should stick to pure English lavender essential oil if at all possible. Pure lavender can be used directly on hemorrhoids as it is gentle on the skin.

Lavender is a versatile essential oil with a wide array of uses. Its soothing properties make it ideal for treating burns, while its ability to calm is great to de-stress and help relax before bed. It's a natural emollient for wounds, anti-oxidant, anti-microbial, anti-allergenic and anti-inflammatory. Lavender essential oil is also used to treat depression, upset stomachs, sore muscles, headaches, insomnia, eczema and psoriasis. It also helps with seasonal sniffles, maintains normal blood pressure levels and supports healthy female cycles.

While lavender is considered safe for use on adults, it may cause skin irritation. When ingested, it may cause headaches, constipation and an increased appetite. According to the U.S. National Library of Medicine, lavender is possibly unsafe for boys who have not reached puberty. This is because lavender essential oil can disrupt the normal hormones in the body.

For those of you that are interested I have created a very in depth book exclusively about Lavender essential oil. It is around 100 pages and contains all the information you could possible need about this one oil. It includes a further 40 recipes to the 100+ in this book. To find it type this link into your web browser:

http://www.amazon.com/dp/B00WTBTHPC. Be aware that they are zeroes and not the letter O!

Peppermint (Mentha piperita)

One of the main therapeutic qualities of peppermint (*Mentha piperita*) is as an agent to relieve stomach complaints. As an essential oil, this can be achieved by massaging a few diluted drops into the skin of the abdomen. Additionally, peppermint can be massaged into fatigued muscles to provide pain relief (thanks to the soothing menthol that the plant contains). Peppermint oil can also be applied to the temples to relieve headaches, to reinvigorate, and to clear nasal passages when inhaled. Additionally, peppermint is believed to trigger part of the brain responsible for feeling 'fullness' after eating; therefore, peppermint may be used to induce this sensation by being inhaled. Concentrated amounts of therapeutic grade peppermint oil should be used with caution as it is especially potent and can irritate the skin of some users.

For thousands of years, peppermint has been revered for its abundance of medicinal properties. Because of its pleasant taste, peppermint is a popular flavoring for drinks and foods, and is also a common choice for fragrances. The ancient Egyptians cultivated and used the leaves of peppermint for indigestion, while the ancient Greeks and Romans used it to soothe stomach pains. In the 18th century, Europeans used it for menstrual disorders and various stomach ailments. The health benefits of peppermint are so well known that it has been verified by many scientific trials and research.

Peppermint essential oil has several health benefits and dietary uses. It is an all-natural remedy for coughing symptoms and the common cold. Its soothing effect can help to calm certain ailments associated with the common cold. It also has antioxidant and anti-microbial qualities, and helps to promote a strong immune system. Peppermint oil has shown to have the ability to reduce inflammation in the throat and mouth. This means that it can be used to treat sinus infections and inflammations.

Nausea and painful cramps are a few of the menstrual symptoms that can be eased with peppermint. This is because it acts as a natural muscle relaxer to reduce the pain of cramps.

The menthol naturally found in peppermint is a common ingredient in over-the-counter pain relievers. It is used to treat toothaches, headaches, joint inflammation, nerve pain, and general muscle pains and body aches.

When diluted properly with carrier oils, peppermint essential oil can help alleviate various skin problems, such as dry skin and rashes. It can also soothe dry and oily scalps when used as a hair rinse. Peppermint herbal supplements are a common remedy for infections, allergic rashes, itchiness and bacterial infections. Peppermint is also a well-known energy booster and stress reducer. Inhaling peppermint will increase energy levels, while clearing the mind and reducing restlessness and anxiety.

While not enough scientific evidence is yet available to support the claim, some people use peppermint essential oil to treat UTIs, also known as urinary tract infections. This may be because of its antibacterial properties, which can help reduce the frequency and symptoms associated with UTIs.

When used properly, peppermint essential oil is safe for adults. With that said, however, you should always use it with caution. Peppermint contains menthol and doses of menthol over 1 gram can be fatal. Furthermore, peppermint essential oil should not be used on children that are under 30-months of age and direct applications to the chest or nasal area of infants can increase the risk of acute respiratory distress respiratory arrest, apnea, bronchial spasms and laryngeal. People of all ages may experience dizziness, muscle weakness, double vision, nausea and confusion when inhaling large doses of menthol.

Eucalyptus (*Eucalyptus Globulus*)

As the plant genus from which it is derived – *Eucalyptus Globulus* – is native to Australia, the therapeutic oil of Eucalyptus has not enjoyed a long history of use. Yet, eucalyptus is an incredibly dynamic essential oil and is typically one of the first turned to in the practice of aromatherapy due to its versatility. It has anti-inflammatory, antispasmodic, antiseptic, antibacterial, and decongestant properties (to name a few) and can be used for a range of treatments – from lice, to asthma, to mental exhaustion. This is one of the top five essential oils you should keep at hand.

Eucalyptus essential oil is derived from about 500 different eucalyptus species. However, the most common species of eucalyptus used for essential oils are *Eucalyptus polybractea*, *Eucalyptus globulus*, *Eucalyptus radiate* and *Eucalyptus citriodora*. I recommend you search for eucalyptus oil made from the Eucalyptus globulus species.

The Australian aboriginals used eucalyptus to treat fever, colds, body pains and sinus congestions. In the 1880s, surgeons would use eucalyptus essential oil in operations as an anti-septic. In fact, the oil was used in English hospitals toward the end of the century to clean urinary catheters. As the years passed, eucalyptus gained more attention and in 1948 it was officially registered in the United States as a miticide and insecticide.

Eucalyptus essential oil has many uses. A diluted form of the oil can be taken orally to relieve inflammation and pain of the respiratory tract mucous membranes, sinus pain, inflammation, asthma, coughs, bronchitis and respiratory infections. It can also be used as an insect repellent, antiseptic, and natural treatment method for burns, ulcers and wounds.

Eucalyptus oil is a common ingredient in perfumes and cosmetics, and is even found in toothpastes, lozenges, cough drops, mouthwashes, ointments and liniments. Other oils are commonly mixed with it to make it more easily absorbed when applied to the skin. When added to skin products, eucalyptus oil acts like a natural sunscreen.

The antibacterial properties found in eucalyptus helps to treat upper respiratory tract problems associated with pathogenic bacteria and protection against tooth decay caused by bacteria.

Many individuals use eucalyptus essential oil to treat mental exhaustion. This is because the oil has a refreshing and cooling effect, while acting as a stimulant to help alleviate mental sluggishness and exhaustion. It is also used to increase blood flow to the brain and stimulate mental activity. Because of this, it is not uncommon for eucalyptus essential oil to be used aromatically in classrooms.

Made up of over 100 different compounds, the main chemical components of eucalyptus essential oil are b-pinene, a-pinene, 1,8-cineole, a-phellandrene, terpinen-4-ol, limonene, piperitone, epiglobulol, aromadendrene and globulol.

While eucalyptus oil is considered safe for use on adults, it shouldn't be used on babies and children unless otherwise directed by a doctor. Furthermore, no one should take this essential oil orally unless under the direct supervision of a doctor. Taking eucalyptus orally can be toxic if not done so properly.

Lemon (Citrus limon)

One of the most common essential oils due to the ubiquity of the humble lemon tree (*Citrus limon*). The essence of lemon is perhaps best known for its use in the culinary world. However, lemon also has fantastic potential for therapeutic application, due to its powerful cleansing properties. A good source of the antioxidant d-limonene, lemon can be used to refresh and cleanse the skin, to clear the mind of stress and to boost the immune system. It is also effective against plaque, cavities and gingivitis due to its antibacterial qualities and can therefore be used as a mouthwash.

The benefits of lemon have been well-known throughout history. In fact, writer Maude Grieve wrote a book on herbal medicine in 1931 that said, "The lemon is the most valuable of all fruit for preserving health." For centuries this oil has been used to lower the acidity level in the body, and in the 1790s, sailors of the Royal Navy were given lemon oil to combat scurvy and treat vitamin deficiencies. Lemon essential oil has been widely used for centuries as a way to reduce wrinkles, cleanse the skin and combat acne. Lemon oil can even be used as a disinfectant in homemade cleaners.

Lemon oil is often used in aromatherapy because of its delightful aroma, and cleansing and uplifting properties. When diffused, it can help eliminate negative emotions and replace them with a more pure, cheerful and fresh outlook. Lemon has also shown to dispel psychological heaviness and mental fatigue. When inhaled, lemon essential oil can increase awareness and concentration. During a Japanese study, lemon oil was diffused in a busy office, and during this time the amount of typing errors actually decreased by 54-percent.

The detoxifying and astringent nature of lemon oil makes it great for treating blemishes caused by oily skin. And its rejuvenating properties means it will brighten listless and dull skin. In fact, some people place slices of lemon on freckles to lighten their appearance.

The active compounds in lemon oil are Alpha-pinene, Alpha-terpinene, Beta-bisabolene, Beta-Pinene. Camphene, Myrcene, Linalool, Limonene, Neral, Nerol, Sabinene and Trans-a-bergamotene.

Lemon essential oil is a powerful antiseptic and astringent, which means it can cause skin irritation to those with sensitive skin. Because of this, lemon oil should never be applied to the skin undiluted. Furthermore, lemon oil contains compounds that lead to photosensitivity, which, when in the presence of sunlight, can increase the chance of skin damage and burns. That is why it is important to never use lemon essential oil within 12 hours of coming in contact with sunlight.

Chamomile (Anthemis nobilis) and (Matricaria chamomilla)

Essence of chamomile is available in two main varieties: one derived from the Roman Chamomile (*Anthemis nobilis)*, the other from German Chamomile (*Matricaria chamomilla*). Though both are quite similar and have a range of common general applications, each possesses certain specific therapeutic qualities. The former is particularly useful as a calming agent, while the latter has powerful anti-inflammatory properties. Both varieties can be used: for detoxification; as an antidepressant; for issues relating to circulation; and for the topical treatment of scars and other blemishes on the skin.

Despite the name, Roman chamomile wasn't cultivated in that area until the 16th century when it arrived via Britain. Since then, however, it has been used as a medicinal plant. Since the first century, German chamomile has been used to treat digestive problems and is even gentle enough for children. The Egyptians worshiped chamomile above all the other herbs and even dedicated it to the sun. There are even hieroglyphic records that show chamomile was used for, at the very least, 2,000 years cosmetically. The noblewomen of Egypt used the crushed chamomile petals on their skin. Physicians in Greece would prescribe chamomile to treat female disorders and fevers, while the herb was added as one of the nine sacred herbs in the ancient Anglo-Saxon manuscript "Lacnunga". The doctors in England and a Virginian colony would keep chamomile on hand in their medical bags. The herb was so highly valued that in some areas in Eastern Europe, such as Romania, children were asked to bring chamomile to school for collection campaigns run by the government.

The key components in Roman chamomile include flavonoids, cyanogenic glycosides, coumarins, phenolic acids, sesquiterpene lactones, salicylates, valerianic acid, tannins and volatile oil, while the key components in German chamomile include bitter glycosides, coumarins, chamazulene, cyanogenic glycosides, salicylates flavonoids, valerianic acid, tannins and volatile oil. As you may notice there are some major differences in the components of each of the oils!

Roman chamomile is a well-known antispasmodic, antiseptic, anti-inflammatory, digestive stimulant, antiallergic, muscle relaxant, mild analgesic and sedative. German chamomile has anti-inflammatory, antiallergenic, antispasmodic, digestive, carminative, relaxant, mild bitter and sedative properties.

While Roman chamomile and German chamomile are often used interchangeably, there are some key differences between the two. Roman chamomile, for example, has much more bitter action than German chamomile. Both varieties, however, have good antibiotic and antiseptic properties. This means they can help eliminate infections and kill intestinal worms. When applied to the hair, both types of chamomile will kill mites and lice.

Both Roman and German chamomile have shown to be an effective oil against depression. These herbs can eliminate feelings of disappointment, sadness, sluggishness and depression, while increase the feelings of happiness and raise spirits.

Roman chamomile has shown to be effective in calming anger, irritation and annoyance, even in small children. German chamomile, however, is effective for curing inflammation, especially when it occurs in the urinary or digestive system. Both varieties curb blood vessel swelling and help to reduce blood pressure.

You shouldn't take chamomile essential oil internally, except under the care of a doctor. People allergic to ragweed and its relatives, chrysanthemums and aster should avoid all forms of chamomile as it could bring on hives and symptoms associated with hay fever. Furthermore, chamomile oil may cause uterine stimulation and pregnant women should avoid using it. While not too common, chamomile essential oil may cause contact dermatitis in some users.

Frankincense (Boswellia carteria.)

Frankincense has a rich history of use as an essential oil, having been used notably as a holy anointing oil in various religions. Extracted from the resin of the frankincense tree (*Boswellia carteri*), it was also used by Ancient Egyptians in facemasks for rejuvenation. The active ingredients in this oil have a strong connection with mental alertness and focus, and can be applied topically to improve concentration. Additionally, frankincense may also be used as an anti-aging agent and to revitalize dry skin, and can also be useful for maintaining uterine health.

Frankincense essential oil is derived from the Boswellia genus tree, with *Boswellia carteria* and *Boswellia sacra* being the two most common.

Traditionally, frankincense was burned for incense, and charred and ground into a powder. This powder was then used as an eyeliner for the ancient Egyptians. In the Middle East, frankincense essential oil has long been revered for its use in religious ceremonies and as an anointing oil.

When used in aromatherapy, frankincense essential oil is an effective sedative that promotes relaxation, feelings of mental peace and satisfaction. It also helps to relieve stress, anger and anxiety.

Frankincense oil has shown to promote the regeneration of healthy cells, while helping to keep tissues and existing cells healthy. This essential oil is also used to reverse the signs of aging, reduce the appearance of scars and stretch marks, treat dry skin and for overall skin health. Frankincense essential oil also has astringent properties that helps:

- Stop bleeding wounds

- Strengthen hair roots and gums

- Speed up the healing of insect bites, cuts, boils and acne

Scientists at Cardiff University found that frankincense essential oil can help to inhibit the production of inflammatory molecules. This helps to prevent the cartilage tissue from breaking down, thus treating arthritis and rheumatoid arthritis.

Frankincense oil is also known for its ability to break up phlegm that is in the lungs and respiratory tract. Because of this, the oil can be used to treat colds, respiratory disorders and bronchitis-related congestion. Frankincense essential oil is good for treating digestive disorders as it helps to speed up gastric juice secretion, bile and acids, thus stimulating the food to move properly through the intestines.

Since frankincense essential oil has antiseptic properties, it can be used to prevent cavities, mouth sores, toothaches, bad breath and other infections. Furthermore, frankincense oil helps to regulate the production of estrogen in women, while reducing the chance of post-menopause uterus tumor or cyst formation. It also is effective at regulating the menstrual cycle of premenopausal women.

While no hard scientific research is available at the moment, frankincense essential oil is being studied for its possible potential as a cancer treatment. An agent naturally found in the oil has been observed by scientists to stop cancer from spreading and cause the cancerous cells to close down.

Frankincense is generally considered safe for use in adults, but you should consider performing a spot test to determine any sensitivity when using this oil for the first time. While some adults can take frankincense oil internally, children ages six years and below should never ingest the oil. Frankincense essential oil is not recommended for individuals pregnant or nursing because it acts as an emenagogue that can induce menstruation.

Side effects of frankincense essential oil are typically not severe, but, in rare cases, it can cause gastrointestinal distress, stomach pain, skin rashes, hyperacidity and nausea. It can also have a blood thinning effect and may increase the chance of abnormal bleeding in individuals who are taking anticoagulant medication or have a bleeding disorder.

Geranium (Pelargonium Odorantissimum)

Geranium is obtained from the leaves and stems of *Pelargonium Odorantissimum*. With a very similar scent to rose, essence of geranium can be used to regenerate damaged tissues, thanks to its cytophylactic properties (which encourages the recycling of dead cells and the production of new ones). As such it can be applied to treat, for example, cuts, bruises, dermatitis, eczema and ulcers. Additionally, it is also a hemostatic compound, meaning it can reduce the incidence and profuseness of bleeding. Essence of geranium is also a good treatment for stress and symptoms of PMS.

The uses of geranium can be traced as far back as the ancient Egyptians, who would use the oil to treat cancerous tumors. In the late 17th century, geranium was brought to Europe and, in the Victorian era, became quite popular. Geranium leaves were placed on dining tables in formal settings and used as finger bowls. During this era, potted geranium plants were placed on tables in the parlor so people could easily obtain a fresh sprig.

Geranium essential oil has various health benefits. It has tonic, deodorant, astringent, diuretic, hemostatic, cytophlyactic, cicatrisant, styptic, vulnerary agent and vermifuge properties.

It is commonly used in aromatherapy because of its ability to relieve depression and stress, balance hormones, reduce irritation and inflammation, alleviate symptoms of menopause, improve skin health, boost kidney health, improve circulation, reduce blood pressure and promote dental health.

Geranium essential oil has antioxidant, antibacterial and antifungal properties. Because of this it can help inhibit the growth of bacterial strains *Yersinia enterolitica* and *Brevibacterium linens*, and one of the most common fungal species *Aspergillus niger*. Geranium oil can also help to prevent bacterial infections. Geranium essential oil also works as a deodorant that can prevent body odor because of its antibacterial properties.

The astringent properties naturally found in geranium essential oil causes skin, tissue, blood vessels, hums, intestines and muscles to contract. This means that the oil can help prevent skin problems, such as wrinkling and sagging, while giving your muscles a more toned appearance. Furthermore, because geranium essential oil improves blood circulation directly below the skin surface and helps to promote proper distribution of melanin, it can help reduce or eliminate the appearance of dark spots and scars.

Geranium essential oil promotes the detoxification process by increasing urination. This will help to remove toxins from the body, while also helping to inhibit the buildup of excess gas in intestines and promote healthy digestive functions. Geranium essential oil also promotes blood clotting, which can speed up the wound healing process, and prevents toxins from reaching the bloodstream via the open wound.

While it is rare, geranium essential oil may have sensitizing effects and it should never be applied directly to the skin without first diluting it in a carrier oil or water. Geranium oil should never be used by pregnant women or nursing mothers as it can influence certain hormone secretions. Furthermore, avoid using geranium essential oil on babies and children as it can be harmful to their delicate skin. And extreme caution should be taken when using this oil around children's noses as it can lead to toxicity.

Ginger (Zingiber officinale)

Like peppermint, ginger (*Zingiber officinale*) can be used very effectively in the treatment of symptoms related to the digestive tract. Complaints such as nausea, heartburn and indigestion may be alleviated with the aid of this essential oil. Additionally, the zesty aroma of ginger can have an energizing effect and increase alertness, while topical application of the oil can improve circulation and alleviate symptoms associated with arthritis.

Ginger is a spicy, energizing and warm oil that has been used for thousands of years for its culinary and medicinal properties. When ginger was exported to the Roman Empire by the Arab traders, it quickly became a popular trade and was even used in sweets. Ginger and black pepper were a commonly traded spice in the 13th and 14th century. It was so desired that one pound of ginger would be traded for one sheep.

Ginger essential oil has many benefits, which are attributed to its stimulating, anti-inflammatory, antiseptic, digestive, analgesic, expectorant and carminative properties. The carminative and antiseptic properties make ginger essential oil a good treatment for food poisoning, as well as bacterial dysentery and intestinal infections.

Ginger is also good for bowel and stomach-related problems. It helps to promote healthy digestion and is a natural remedy for indigestion, spasms, flatulence and dyspepsia. Ginger has also shown to increase appetite, which can be beneficial for individuals trying to gain weight for health reasons. Ginger can also reduce pain. Prostaglandins are compounds associated with pain. And ginger – both ginger root and ginger oil – can help reduce these compounds, thus controlling pain.

Ginger essential oil has shown to be useful at treating respiratory problems. It can help relieve and treat asthma, flu, coughs, bronchitis and breathlessness. In fact, consuming fresh ginger, such as in a tea, can help remove mucus from the lungs and throat.

Regular use of ginger oil can help reduce the chance of blood clots and arteriosclerosis, while decreasing the levels of blood cholesterol in the blood. Furthermore, a study found that ginger essential oil can help repel the mosquito species known to be the primary carrier of malaria and yellow fever in India.

People who have a sensitivity to ginger root should never use ginger essential oil. Ginger essential oil is generally considered safe, and is usually non-irritating and non-toxic. However, people with sensitive skin may experience an unpleasant reaction to the essential oil. You can avoid any ill reaction by first testing the ginger essential oil on a small patch of skin before use. If you develop an allergic reaction, discontinue use immediately. If, however, no adverse reaction occurs, continue to use as desired.

Despite its relatively safe nature, ginger essential oil should always be diluted with a carrier oil. Furthermore, ginger oil may have a phototoxic effect, so you shouldn't apply it to any skin that will experience sunlight exposure within 24 hours of the application.

While ginger essential oil has been shown to be useful for morning sickness, pregnant women should exercise extreme caution when using it. In fact, pregnant women should only use ginger essential oil when under the supervision of their healthcare provider. Also, the use of ginger essential oil on babies and young children should be avoided.

The side effects of ginger essential oil are typically not serious and include sores in the mouth, skin rashes when applied topically, heartburn and nausea. To help reduce the chance of developing any side effects, consult with your doctor. He or she will be able to tell you if the essential oil will react badly with any medications you are currently taking.

Neroli (Citrus aurantium)

Although most famous for its use in *eau de cologne* (and possibly as one of the closely guarded secret ingredients in Coca-Cola!), essence of neroli also has a range of therapeutic applications. Derived from the blossom of bitter orange (*Citrus aurantium),* neroli can be used therapeutically as a powerful anti-depressant, against bacterial and viral infections of the gut, to treat skin infections, to protect against colds and flus, and even as an aphrodisiac!

In the mid-1500s, the bitter orange tree was brought to St. Augustine, Florida by the Spaniards. In Florida, bitter orange thrived and, by 1763, was exported. The oil extracted from the bitter orange tree was named after the 16th century Princess of Nerola, Italy because she introduced it to Italy and loved the scent of the orange blossoms. Napoleon Bonaparte – the French military leader – and the Duchess Marie Antoinette both loved neroli essential oil and used it daily as an aftershave and fragrance.

Throughout ancient times, neroli essential oil was commonly used to relieve fever, banish nervousness and combat the plague. Ancient Egyptian priestesses and priests used this essential oil to heal their mind, spirit and body. The pleasant scent of neroli oil has made it a widely popular ingredient in fragrances and perfumes. The well-known perfume from Cologne Germany – Eau-de-Cologne – used neroli oil as its main ingredient.

When applied topically, neroli essential oil can help keep skin healthy, regenerate skin elasticity, banish acne, help to heal broken capillaries, reduce the appearance of scars and prevent stretch marks. When used in aromatherapy, neroli essential oil is used for its relaxing and calming scent, and even acts as a natural tranquilizer that can help relieve insomnia, treat stress-related depression, heart palpitations and alleviate anxiety. Diffused, the essential oil can help treat various digestive issues, like diarrhea, intestinal spasms, dyspepsia and colitis. The pleasant aroma of neroli essential oil works well as a deodorant to keep foul odors at bay. Furthermore, when diffused or sprayed into the area, it can kill toxins and germs.

Neroli essential oil has various health-promoting and beneficial aspects attributed to its disinfectant, bactericidal, antiseptic, antidepressant, sedative and antispasmoic properties.

In emergency situations, neroli essential oil can be a natural substitute for anti-tetanus by protecting wounds from infections. Keep in mind, however, that neroli essential oil shouldn't replace a trip to the doctor's for a proper tetanus shot and should, instead, be used to hold off infections until the wound can be properly treated by a physician.

Neroli essential oil can help kill bacteria that leads to food poisoning, cholera and typhoid, as well as treating bacteria-caused skin conditions. This essential oil is also a well-known tonic that promotes healthy metabolism, acts as a support for immune system and proper circulation.

When used in moderation, neroli essential oil is not known to be toxic. You should, however, only use the oil when it is diluted with a carrier oil or water. Furthermore, women who are pregnant or breastfeeding, as well as children, shouldn't use neroli essential oil unless advised to by a doctor.

Neroli essential oil may cause mild to moderate side effects, such as headaches, nausea and uneasiness. Also, since neroli oil has natural sedative properties, it shouldn't be used when you need to stay alert and concentrate, such as when driving or operating machinery.

Patchouli (Pogostemon cablin)

Native to South East Asia, the oil of the patchouli plant (*Pogostemon cablin*) is primarily used in issues relating to skincare. Subsequently, it can be used to treat conditions such as acne, eczema, dandruff, dermatitis, and cracked and dry skin. It can also be used to prevent the skin from aging and as a cosmetic treatment to reduce the appearance of scarring. Patchouli also has positive indications for the treatment of stress related issues, such as tension, insomnia and anxiety.

For some people the smell of patchouli essential oil often brings to mind the hippie era that occurred in the' 60s and '70s. This oil, however, has a wealth of beneficial properties that go beyond the pleasant scent. For thousands of years, patchouli has been used and was considered very valuable. The European traders would exchange one pound of the plant for a pound of gold. In ancient Roma, patchouli was used as an appetite stimulant. In ancient Egypt, King Tut arranged for ten gallons of patchouli essential oil to be buried with him after he died.

In Japan, China and Malaysia, patchouli essential oil has been long used in traditional medicine. It is used to treat a wide array of hair and skin problems, including dry and/or chapped skin, acne, eczema, dermatitis, oily scalp and dandruff. It is also used to reduce the appearance of scars, to promote wound healing and increase sexual desire.

Dating back to India in the 19th century, patchouli essential oil has been used as a fabric fragrance. In fact, manufacturers would use the oil as moth repellent for the exported fabrics. Patchouli oil is still used today as a fragrance ingredient in personal care and skin products, paper towels, laundry detergents and air fresheners. When used in aromatherapy, patchouli essential oil helps relieve stress, depression and anxiety.

The health benefits of patchouli oil can be attributed to its anti-inflammatory, astringent, antidepressant, antiseptic, cytophylactic and diuretic properties. It is also an effective insecticide, sedative and deodorant.

Patchouli essential oil is known to soothe irritation and inflammation, including arthritis, gout and other inflammation-related conditions. Patchouli oil also inhibits fungal growth and can provide protection against athlete's foot. For colds and flu, patchouli essential oil bolsters the immune system to help prevent tonsillitis, colds and influenza. It will also help to fight infections that lead to fever, whilst reducing the body temperature. Patchouli essential oil has long been thought of as a tonic that promotes overall wellbeing in the liver, intestines and stomach.

When inhaled or applied topically, patchouli essential oil is generally considered safe. It mixes well with cedarwood, rose, lavender, clary sage, geranium, frankincense and ylang-ylang essential oil. Despite its relatively safe nature, people with sensitive skin may experience a reaction to patchouli oil. Furthermore, you should keep the oil from having direct contact with the nose, eyes and ears.

I recommend that pregnant women stay away from patchouli essential oil during the first trimester of their pregnancy. Please consult with your doctor before using patchouli essential oil if pregnant or nursing.

When used in large amounts, patchouli essential oil can have a strong sedative effect and cause overstimulation. It has also shown to cause appetite loss and photosensitivity. Individuals who are recovering from sickness or who are suffering with an eating disorder should avoid using patchouli essential oil unless otherwise directed to do so by their physician.

Rose (Rosa damascene)

The delightfully scented essence of rose (*Rosa damascene*) is another incredibly versatile essential oil. Its remarkably wide range of applications include: use as an antibacterial and antiseptic agent to protect against external and internal infections; use as an antidepressant, confidence booster and nerve tonic; aiding to induce menstruation and boost libido; revitalization of skin, improving texture and appearance; and use as an agent to purify the blood and decrease the incidence of bleeding.

Throughout the years, roses have been considered one of, if not the most, beautiful and revered flower. This plant has even become an integral part of numerous legends, legacies, stories and myths. Very few people, however, know the medicinal benefits provided by roses and only see the plant for its beautiful blooms. The rose and its essential oil has antidepressant, antiseptic, antiviral, antiphlogistic, antispasmodic, astringent, aphrodisiac, bactericidal, cicatrisant, emenagogue, hepatic, cholagogue, depurative, haemostatic, nervine, uterine, laxative and stomachic properties.

As an antidepressant, rose essential oil boosts mental strength, self-esteem and confidence, while fighting depression and relieving anxiety. When used in aromatherapy, rose essential oil increases positive feelings and thoughts – such as hope, joy and happiness – and spiritual relaxation. Since rose oil is a natural antiphogistic, it can reduce high fevers and treat inflammation caused by microbial infection, dehydration, indigestion and ingesting poisonous materials.

Rose essential oil is an antiseptic that can treat wounds and help prevent them from developing an infection or becoming septic. And its antispasmodic properties relieve spasms in the intestines and respiratory system. Rose oil is a natural antiviral agent that can help shield you from various types of viruses and viral infections.

When used as an aphrodisiac, rose essential oil can boost the libido and improve sex life. It also reduces the symptoms associated with frigidity, erectile dysfunction, sexual dysfunction and general disinterest in any type of sexual activities. The astringent properties of rose oil make it invaluable for strengthening hair roots and gums, while toning skin, intestines and blood vessels. This means that rose oil helps to protect against hair and teeth loss, loss of firmness in the muscles and wrinkles.

Rose essential oil is an effective bactericidal that has been used to treat food poisoning, diarrhea, typhoid, cholera and various other conditions caused by bacteria. It can also treat internal bacterial infections, such as those found in the intestines, stomach, urinary tract and colon. Rose oil also has depurative properties that help to neutralize and remove toxins from the body. Often, once the blood is toxin free and purified, the development of ulcers, rashes, boils and other skin disease reduces. Rose essential oil is known as a natural laxative that helps clear the bowels, while removing toxins from the body.

Rose oil can be useful for individuals who are experiencing hemorrhaging after a surgery or injury. The hemostatic properties of this essential oil helps speed up coagulation and clotting of blood, thus stopping excessive bleeding. Rose essential oil also has hepatic properties that is good for liver health. It promotes a healthy liver that functions properly and is protected against infections. Rose oil can also help treat ulcers and the excessive flow of acids and bile.

When used in the recommended dosages, rose essential oil is relatively safe. However, the strong aroma of rose oil can actually cause headaches when used in high concentration. In addition, rose essential oil is an emenagogue and should be avoided during pregnancy since it can cause a miscarriage.

Rosemary (Rosmarinus officinalis)

Rosemary essence has enjoyed a prominent place in the essential oil family since Roman times, when it was used frequently in religious ceremonies, food preparation, cosmetics and healthcare. Today, it is equally as used and useful. Rosemary (*Rosmarinus officinalis*) has long been associated with memory, and can be used to remedy both mental fatigue and forgetfulness. It also provides good effect for stress and pain relief, indigestion, clear skin and stronger, healthier hair. Recent studies suggest that rosemary can be effective in treating the herpes simplex virus, which can build up a resistance to treatment with regular antiviral medication over time.

Rosemary has long been coveted and rumor has it that the Virgin Mary would, when resting, spread her blue cloak over a blooming rosemary bush, which caused the white flowers to turn blue. Because of this, the rosemary bush became known as the Rose of Mary. The Hebrews, Egyptians, Romans and Greeks considered rosemary to be sacred, and, in the Middle Ages it was used to protect against the plague and ward off evil spirits.

Paracelsus, a 16th-century German-Swiss botanist and physician who was a major contributor to herbal medicine, favorited rosemary because of its many health benefits. Paracelsus valued rosemary essential oil because of the oil's ability to strengthen the entire body and heal sensitive organs, such as the heart, brain and liver.

Rosemary essential oil is known for its antibacterial, anti-catarrhal, anticancer, anti-infection, antifungal, anti-inflammatory, expectorant, antioxidant and analgesic properties.

When used in aromatherapy, rosemary essential oil has shown to decrease cortisol levels, which is a hormone that the body releases in response to stress. A study conducted in 2007 that inhaling rosemary essential oil for five minutes reduces cortisol levels significantly and decreases chronic stress. In the same study, the antioxidant properties of rosemary essential oil were found to help boost immune systems.

Stress isn't the only problem that diffused rosemary essential oil can treat. Anxiety and respiratory problems can also be relieved through aromatherapy when using rosemary essential oil.

Individuals often use rosemary essential oil for relieving stomach cramps, flatulence and bloating. It has also been shown to stimulate appetite. Furthermore, research shows that rosemary essential oil has the ability to detoxify the liver and promote healthy digestion.

Rosemary essential oil is revered for its pain relieving ability, which can help relieve muscle pains, arthritis and headaches. The anti-inflammatory properties of rosemary oil makes it useful for addressing pain associated with joint aches and sprains.

While rosemary essential oil is safe when properly used for its intended purposes, it should always be diluted with a carrier oil if applied topically. Women who are pregnant and/or breastfeeding should avoid using rosemary oil since it can have a negative effect on the fetus and increase the chance of a miscarriage, and it should not be used on children unless advised to do so by a doctor. Furthermore, you must remember that using rosemary essential oil as a treatment of chronic diseases – such as Alzheimer's or depression – without being under the supervision of a physician could have serious consequences.

Tea Tree (Melaleuca alternifolia)

Tea tree oil is extracted from the twigs and leaves of *Melaleuca alternifolia* (which is distinct from the tea plant from which the beverage is brewed). Like eucalyptus, the tea tree is native to Australia, and also like eucalyptus, it has a huge range of therapeutic applications. Tea tree oil has a range of important therapeutic properties as it is antibacterial, antiviral, antiseptic, antimicrobial, a fungicide, a stimulant, an expectorant and an insecticide! Tea tree oil can be used to successfully treat most topical infections and diseases. Due to the sheer multitude of its potential applications, tea tree is a must have essential oil. (*N.B. Tea tree oil should never be ingested as it is poisonous! Please only use as an external treatment*).

In the 1770s, Lieutenant James Cook, a British explorer, found native Australians brewing a tea made with the leaves from the melaleuca tree. He later would brew his own tea using the leaves to prevent his crew from getting scurvy. The aboriginal communities in Australia have long used tea tree to treat, cure and prevent various skin conditions. It wasn't until the 1920s, when an Australian state government chemist named Arthur Penfold published a serious of papers, that the wide array of benefits that tea tree oil has become widely known.

The antibacterial, antiviral and antifungal properties make tea tree oil a long valued essential oil. Surgery and dentistry used tea tree oil in the '20s to clean wounds and help prevent infections. In recent years, the use of tea tree oil has surged and it is even a popular ingredient in shampoos, soaps, lotions and various other personal care products.

When compared to benzoyl peroxide, a common ingredient in acne medicine, tea tree oil has a similar if not better effect on acne. While the onset of action was slower with tea tree oil, there were fewer side effects than benzoyl peroxide.

In 2004, a study conducted by the National Center for Complementary and Alternative Medicine found that tea tree oil could be used to treat wounds and severe infections. Tea tree oil can also be effectively used to treat fungal infections, such as toenail onychomycosis. When diffused and used in aromatherapy, tea tree essential oil helps to relieve stuffy nose, head congestion, chest congestion and other symptoms associated with flu and colds.

Tea tree oil is considered safe as long as it is applied topically and NOT ingested. Keep in mind, however, that tea tree oil may cause mild skin irritation in some people. If this is your first time using tea tree oil, consider performing a test using a low concentrated dose on your skin. This will allow you to determine your tolerance of the oil. If after 24 hours, no reverse effects have occurred, continue as desired. However, if you notice an allergic reaction, discontinue use immediately.

The National Center for Complementary and Alternative Medicine recommends that you use fresh tea tree oil and avoid oxidized oil, which is oil that has been exposed to air. Oxidized tea tree oil can trigger allergies more than fresh oil. Furthermore, you should use tea tree oil only when it has been diluted with a carrier oil, or when used in cream, lotions and gels.

Tea tree oil contains 1,8-cineole, which is a skin irritant that can cause allergic reactions in some people. These reactions are typically mild rashes that itch, but blistering can also occur. Serious allergic reactions include swelling of the throat and dizziness. Individuals who are allergic to eucalyptols should avoid using tea tree oil.

Tea tree essential oil has also shown to pose a threat to pets when ingested. Large amounts of undiluted oil applied to the skin of dogs and cats can lead to hypersensitive reaction. To keep your pets safe, avoid using this essential oil unless directed to do so by a trusted veterinarian.

Ylang Ylang (Cananga odorata).

Essence of ylang ylang is obtained from the steam distillation of flowers from the ylang ylang tree (*Cananga odorata*). This extract has great potential for cosmetic use as its use can result in both thick hair and smooth skin. It is also effective for lowering blood pressure and strengthening the nervous system. Additionally, it holds the unique characteristic of being an effective treatment for seborrhea, an acute and chronic form of eczema which is caused by irregular function of the sebaceous glands. Finally, ylang ylang has also shown effectiveness in providing relief from stress and anxiety.

The history of ylang ylang essential oil is not well known. In fact, it wasn't until recently that this essential oil become widely available. Thanks to a flood of advertisements, ylang ylang essential oil is getting the recognition it deserves. Ylang ylang has antidepressant, antiseptic, hypotensive, antiseborrhoeic, nervine, sedative and aphrodisiac properties, thus making this essential oil a popular and useful tool.

One of ylang ylang's oldest known medicinal uses is as an antidepressant. Not only does this essential oil fight depression, but it also relaxes the soul and body and keeps chronic stress, sadness and anxiety at bay. It replaces these unpleasant feelings with hope and joy. Ylang ylang has even shown to help treat individuals who have acute depression that occurs after an accident or shock as well as for those people dealing with a nervous breakdown.

Ylang ylang essential oil is a powerful antiseptic that can help keep abrasions, burns and cuts from becoming septic or tetanus. Its ability to disinfect wounds and inhibit microbial growth goes a long way to preventing virus, fungus and bacteria, while speeding up the healing process.

Ylang ylang essential oil has proven to lower blood pressure that can occur in people young and old. This comes in handy especially since the prescription blood pressure medication can come with some serious and potentially dangerous side effects. Keep in mind, however, that no essential oil should be used as a substitute for professional medical advice and you should always speak to your doctor before starting any essential oil.

When dealing with professional stress, overloaded at work or depression, your sex drive can take a huge hit. Diffusing ylang ylang essential oil in your home can help improve sexual life and libido.

The calming and sedative properties of ylang ylang essential oil helps to relieve anxiety, stress, anxiety and anger, while bringing on a relaxed feeling. It has also been shown to help boost nervous systems.

Ylang ylang essential oil may be relatively new compared to other essential oils but with all the benefits it provides, it holds its own. In fact, ylang ylang oil can cure infections in the colon, stomach, urinary tract and intestines. It also can treat fatigue, insomnia and other conditions related to stress while acting as a wonderful moisturizer for dry skin.

Ylang ylang essential oil is consider relatively safe, however, some individuals have experienced sensitivity, headaches and nausea when using the oil in excess. Sticking to the recommended does will help prevent any side effects from occurring.

Sandalwood (Santalum spp.)

Essence of sandalwood is extracted from the matured wood of the sandalwood tree, with Indian (*Santalum album*), Hawaiian (*Santalum ellipticum*) and Australian (*Santalum spicatum*) varieties available. Due to the prevalence of sandalwood in India, it has a long history of use in rituals and ceremonies at all stages of life there. Sandalwood has a great range of health related benefits, which include reducing high blood pressure and bad cholesterol, anti-inflammatory and anti-aging properties, providing a boost to immunity and aiding memory and concentration. Additionally, sandalwood can be used to treat urinary tract infections, prevent flatulence and aid in weight loss.

For over four thousand years, sandalwood essential oil has been used for its many health benefits and exotic scent. It is a common ingredient in personal care products, cosmetics, fragrances, and spiritual/meditative practices. The woody, pleasant scent is lingering yet subtle, and can create a calm, harmonizing effect that helps to reduce confusion and tension. Ancient Egypt, Rome and Greece would commonly use sandalwood for various purposes. In fact, temples were often built using sandalwood, as well as caskets and furniture.

Sandalwood has now become a popular oil used in yoga practices. It is diffused to treat daily stress, anxiety, depression, chronic illness and fear. But that isn't all sandalwood oil is used for. When used in skincare, it relieves inflammation, itching and dry, dehydrated skin. It can be used to treat scar tissue, eczema, rashes, psoriasis, dandruff and acne. Sandalwood essential oil is also used as a remedy for respiratory concerns.

The anti-inflammatory properties of sandalwood have a cooling effect on digestive, circulatory, excretory, brain and nervous systems. It has also shown to soothe skin irritation, inflammation and cure infections, while promoting a cool, fresh feeling. Since sandalwood is an antispasmodic, it can help relax nerves, blood vessels and muscles. The astringent properties naturally found in this essential oil mean it can tighten skin and provide better muscle strength. In addition, sandalwood is an expectorant that can help fight infections caused by flu, cold, mumps and cough.

Sandalwood has disinfectant and deodorant properties that can keep small insects and microbes at bay, while relieving body odor. Sandalwood essential oil is also a memory booster. Regular users of this oil have reported better concentration and memory after use.

While sandalwood essential oil is typically consider safe, there are some precautions and warnings you should know before using. Sandalwood oil is not meant for ingesting and should only be used topically or aromatically. When using sandalwood essential oil topically, you should always dilute it in a carrier oil, lotion, soap or various other buffering agents. Women who are breastfeeding and children shouldn't use sandalwood essential oil. Furthermore, some individuals may have an allergic skin reaction when using sandalwood essential oil. People suffering from cancer or liver disorders should not use sandalwood oil unless advised to do so by their doctor.

Despite the fact that sandalwood oil may relax and calm pets, it can be extremely toxic to cats. That is why you should avoid using essential oils without first consulting with a trusted veterinarian.

Cedarwood (Juniperus virginiana)

The essence of cedarwood is extracted through steam distillation of pieces of wood from the cedarwood tree (*Juniperus virginiana*), which is normally found in cold climates. While cedarwood shares some common therapeutic properties with other popular essential oils (such as being an antiseptic, anti-inflammatory, and, like ylang ylang, a treatment for seborrhea), it also has some relatively unique applications. Amongst these, cedarwood acts as an effective stimulant of metabolism, improving general feelings of wellness and encouraging weight loss. Additionally, it acts as a strong natural sedative, with powerful calming and relaxing qualities.

Ancient Egyptians used cedarwood essential oil as an ingredient in perfume and the embalming process, as well as an insect repellant. The Native Americans would burn cedar essential oil for purification and medicinal purposes. The ancient Greeks preserved bodies with cedarwood essential oil because they believed it helped to make the person immortal. In various areas around the world, cedarwood essential oil has been used as an ant, moth and general insect repellent.

The Far East would use cedarwood essential oil as a preserver and as a urinary tract and bronchial infection treatment. It was also used as a popular incense. Tibetans used cedarwood essential oil as medicine and as an incense burned in their temples, which is still used in this manner today.

Cedarwood essential oil has antiseptic, tonic, antiseborrhoeic, antispasmodic, diuretic, expectorant, sedative, astringent, emenagogue, insecticidal and fungicidal properties.

As an antiseptic, cedarwood essential oil helps to prevent wounds from turning septic, while also protecting them against tetanus germs. Several herbal antiseptic creams list cedarwood as a main ingredient in their formulas. The antispasmodic properties of cedarwood essential oil can relieve just about any type of spasm, including those that affect muscles, nerves, intestines, heart and the respiratory system. The soothing properties of this oil can also help individuals who are experiencing restless leg syndrome, asthma, respiratory seizers and various other spasmodic conditions.

Cedarwood essential oil has long been used as a general health tonic that has the ability to simulate metabolism and promote healthy skin, muscles, stomachs, nervous and digestive systems. As a tonic, cedarwood oil boosts the functions of the liver and kidney, which has a direct impact on your overall health and well-being.

The natural astringent properties of cedarwood oil make it useful for treating toothaches while strengthening the grip that gums have on teeth, thus preventing them from falling out. Cedarwood essential oil also works to give you a youthful, firm and fit feeling due to its ability to tighten loose muscles. As a diuretic, cedarwood essential oil can help treat a wide array of ailments such as high blood pressure, urinary tract infections, hypertension, arthritis, obesity, rheumatism, gout and toxins in the blood.

Cedarwood essential oil can help remove phlegm from the lungs and the respiratory tract while eliminating coughs. This is due to its expectorant properties. Furthermore, cedarwood oil can relieve watery, red eyes, headaches and other symptoms associated with colds and coughs.

Cedarwood essential oil naturally soothes and calms, which makes it an effective sedative. When used in aromatherapy, cedarwood essential oil can promote healthy uninterrupted sleep and even treat insomnia. It can also help treat chronic stress, depression and anxiety.

Cedarwood essential oil's main chemical components are cedrol, b-cedrene, a-cedrene, sesquiterpenes, widdrol and thujopsene.

Cedarwood essential oil can be irritating to the skin when used in high concentrations. Young children and pregnant women should avoid this essential oil because of its toxicity. Some countries, such as France, have even restricted the use of cedarwood essential oil because of its neuro toxic and abortive abilities. With that said, cedarwood essential oil is relatively safe if used properly and with care.

Jasmine (Jasminum officinale)

Extracted from the fragrant jasmine blossom (*Jasminum officinale)*, jasmine essential oil shares the distinctive sweet aroma of its source. While it is generally recommended that pregnant and nursing mothers should avoid the use of essential oils, many of the special therapeutic qualities of jasmine are centered on the birthing process or post-natal health of the mother. For example, jasmine can be applied to reduce labor pains in women, and facilitate the birthing process. Additionally, it can also be used to promote lactation, and help women re-adjust to post pregnancy life by encouraging uterine health, encouraging regular menstrual cycles and boosting libido at a time when desire may have waned. (*N.B. Because of the risks associated with exposing children to essential oils, advice on their administration should be sought if used by expectant or new mothers*).

Jasmine has been used for centuries for various reasons and is even the national flower of Pakistan. The flowers, leaves and roots of the jasmine plant have been used for culinary, aromatic, ceremonial and medicinal purposes. In the Indian subcontinent, jasmine is important in certain religious ceremonies and is offered to Lord Vishnu as a sacred offering. Garlands made with the jasmine flower are used for welcoming guests and is a symbol of respect. In Vedic rituals, the sweet smelling jasmine flower is added to hair as ornaments.

Jasmine essential oil was a favorite anointing oil for kings during the time of Lord Buddha, and it was used as a remedy for poisonous stings and bites. Traditional Chinese medicine used jasmine as an aphrodisiac, as well as various other medicinal purposes including treating hepatitis.

When used in aromatherapy, jasmine essential oil can help to sooth nerves and treat depression. It can also promote feelings of optimism, euphoria and confidence, while restoring and revitalizing energy.

In childbirth, jasmine helps to facilitate delivery by strengthening contractions while relieving pain. It also promotes the healthy flow of breast milk and acts as a treatment for post-natal depression.

Jasmine has a calming and soothing nature that has shown useful for treating sexual problems, like frigidity, impotence and premature ejaculation.

The respiratory system can benefit from jasmine essential oil, which helps treat laryngitis and hoarseness, while soothing irritating coughs. It also helps treat sprains, stiff limbs and muscle pain. For skin problems, jasmine essential oil treats, irritated, greasy, sensitive and dry skin, while reducing the appearance of scarring and stretch marks, and increasing elasticity.

The benefits of jasmine essential oil are attributed to its antiseptic, antispasmodic, antidepressant, aphrodisiac, emmenagogue, cicatrisant, sedative, parturient, uterine and galactogogue properties.

While jasmine essential oil is non-irritant, non-toxic and typically non-sensitizing, some individuals may experience an allergic reaction to the oil. Furthermore, women who are pregnant should avoid jasmine essential oil because of its emmenagogue properties. Jasmine essential oil is a deeply relaxing oil and shouldn't be used if you will need to concentrate.

Clove (Syzygium aromaticum)

The oil of clove (*Syzygium aromaticum*) has a sweet, spicy aroma, which is often used in perfumes and soaps. Among clove's many therapeutic properties, it is an antimicrobial, antiseptic, antifungal and antiviral. It can be used to effectively treat ear and eye infections, and can also be used to help treat the problem of premature ejaculation. Clove has also shown to be a potentially effective treatment for diabetes, as it assists with both blood purification and circulation, and thanks to the high concentration of phenol in the spice, helps to control blood sugar levels. (*N.B. As essence of clove is a particularly strong essential oil, it should be used with caution. It should typically always be diluted and applied in small amounts on first usage*).

The aromatic spice known as clove has been used for centuries for its medicinal and seasoning purposes. The ancient Romans and Greeks would use clove essential oil to alleviate bad breath and treat toothaches. Ancient Chinese medicine also used clove essential oil for its oral health benefits. Clove oil is often used as a mouthwash gargle, dental anesthetic, toothache reliever and fighter against throat and mouth infections. In fact, it is not uncommon to see clove listed as an ingredient in dental and pharmaceutical products.

Many of the health benefits of clove essential oil can be traced back to the eugenol content found in the oil. Ninety percent of the oil is eugenol, which is a compound that has anti-inflammatory and antiseptic benefits. Because of the high amount of this compound, clove essential oil is effective against cavities, sore gums, bad breath, dental pain and mouth ulcers. This compound also gives clove essential oil a warming and stimulating property that makes it a favorite among the practitioners of aromatherapy. When diffused, clove essential oil improves blood circulation, lowers the body temperature and stimulates the metabolism. It also promotes digestive health and can even treat indigestion, excess gas, motion sickness and hiccups. Clove essential oil has been shown to reduce mental exhaustion, while relieving stress, anxiety and depression. As if that wasn't enough, diffused clove oil acts as an aphrodisiac and insomnia treatment.

Using clove oil undiluted can cause serious skin problems. That is why it is important to always dilute clove essential oil with a carrier oil before applying it topically. You should also consider performing a skin test to see if you have an allergic reaction. Clove essential oil is considered a dangerous sensitizer in some people. The high concentrations of eugenol that is found in cloves can cause irritation to the mucous membrane, as well as leading to skin problems like dermatitis. In some instances, clove essential oil can cause photosensitivity and you should never use this oil on damaged skin. Despite all the benefits it has to offer, beginners should only use clove essential oil in moderation.

Individuals using aspirin and/or anticoagulants should never use clove essential oil as it may reduce platelet activity. Clove oil also may cause the blood glucose to drastically plummet, therefore diabetics should exercise caution when using clove essential oil. People suffering from kidney or liver disease should also avoid using clove essential oil since it may damage both organs.

Women who are pregnant or nursing should use caution with clove essential oil. It should also be kept away from children as it has the potential to cause intestinal discomfort.

Ingesting clove essential oil undiluted can cause nausea, sore throat, vomiting, seizures and blood problems. It can also cause rashes, itching and shortness of breath. Even though you can use clove essential oil to treat acne, excessive use can lead to skin damage and permanent marks.

Oregano (Oreganum vulgare)

Perhaps most well-known as a herb used to flavor savory dishes, essence of oregano *(Oreganum vulgare)* has also long been a popular essential oil. It was used extensively in Ancient Greece as a disinfectant and antibacterial agent, and also to protect food from bacteria. Like many other essential oils, oregano has obvious antiviral, antifungal, and antibacterial properties. It is also used today as a powerful painkiller, and, thanks to its high levels of antioxidants, can help to ward off some of the effects of aging, including macular degeneration, degenerative nervous system disorders, and certain age related cancers.

The ancient Romans and Greeks used oregano for various medicinal purposes. It was even thought of as a symbol of happiness and used to crown brides and grooms. Oregano essential oil has a wide array of health benefits. It is most notably used for immune and respiratory system health. Furthermore, oregano essential oil can help treat and prevent infections, such as urinary tract infections (UTIs), yeast infections, respiratory infections, parasitic infections and methicillin-resistant staphylococcus aureus infection (MRSA).

Research has shown that oregano essential oil can help prevent food-borne illnesses caused by E. coli, salmonella, listeria and various other pathogens. It is also known to relieve respiratory illnesses and coughs. In addition, oregano essential oil can act as a natural insect repellant to ward off insects, relieve rashes (such as poison ivy) and bug bites, help to heal dandruff, cold sores and other skin conditions, ease sore throats and relieve joint and muscle pain, sprains, cramps and rheumatoid arthritis.

Oregano essential oil is generally considered harmless as long as it's diluted in a carrier oil or water. A good general rule of thumb is to dilute 1 part oregano essential oil with 3 parts carrier oil. If you have never used oregano essential oil, you should perform a spot test to determine if you will have an adverse reaction to the oil. Some individuals may experience mild to moderate stomach upset when ingesting oregano essential oil. Furthermore, people who are allergic to mint, sage, basil, lavender or any other plant in the Lamiaceae family should not use oregano oil.

Oregano essential oil should not be used on infants and children. Pregnant and/or nursing women should also avoid using this oil because it can promote blood circulation in the uterus, thus deteriorating the lining protecting the fetus in the womb. It can also induce menstruation, which can be dangerous for the unborn child.

Grapefruit (Citrus paradisi)

Grapefruit oil, like its other citrus cousins, is often used for its disinfectant properties in cleaning. This quality can also be applied therapeutically to clean wounds and for detox of internal systems. Grapefruit's (*Citrus paradisi)* properties as a super-detox agent are magnified by the fact that it is a lymphatic – this helps ensure the healthy functioning of the body's lymphatic system which is responsible for the removal and filtration of toxic substances from the body. Also, like oregano, grapefruit is rich in antioxidants which help to prevent some of the problems and pathologies associated with aging.

The actual origin and history of grapefruit is rather unknown. Some accounts say that the fruit was bred in Jamaica first. What is known however, is that grapefruit essential oil provides many medicinal benefits. For example, grapefruit has a positive effect on the lymphatic system, which is vital to proper detoxification of the body. Using grapefruit oil will help boost lymph gland activity and help prevent poor circulation, fluid retention, cellulite and allergies. The antimicrobial effects of grapefruit essential oil have been shown in a study to fight bacteria strains, such as Staphylococcus epidermidis, Salmonella thyphimurium, Staphylococcus aureus and Escherichia coli. These antimicrobial properties found in grapefruit essential oil can help prevent and treat infections in cuts and wounds, and can even help eliminate microbes in the excretory system, gut and kidneys.

Grapefruit essential oil is filled with antioxidants and vitamin C, which supports a healthy immune system while fighting free radicals. This means that grapefruit oil helps to prevent oxidation-related damage, including poor hearing, premature aging, macular degeneration and other vision problems and problems with the nervous system. Grapefruit essential oil supports healthy endocrine function and the proper secretion of enzymes and hormones. It also encourages the production of bile and juices to help promote a healthy digestive system.

In aromatherapy, grapefruit essential oil is desired for its antidepressant properties that create an uplifting and relaxing feeling, while stimulating the brain to make you more alert.

Grapefruit essential oil is generally recognized as safe, but it should never be taken internally unless advised to by a doctor. Grapefruit essential oil is also highly concentrated, which means it should always be diluted before use. Some individuals may experience an allergic reaction when the oil is applied topically. Performing a skin patch test will help determine your sensitivity to the oil. As with other citrus essential oils, grapefruit can cause photosensitivity to ultraviolet rays, which would lead to skin problems, such as brown spots, skin discolorations and freckles. That is why it is important to not apply grapefruit essential oil to any skin that will be exposed to the sun for 24 hours after application.

Women who are pregnant or nursing should first speak with their doctor before using grapefruit essential oil. And it shouldn't be used on children of any age since it could harm their sensitive skin. Furthermore, grapefruit essential oil is toxic to cats and should never be used on or around felines.

Lemon Grass (*Cymbopogon citratus*)

The aroma of lemon grass essential oil, as the name suggests is similar to that of lemons. However it is not completely the same, lemon grass essential oil has a milder smell that is sweeter and much less sour. It is dark yellow in color, leaning towards a reddish tinge and is watery in viscosity. It is most commonly known for its use in drinks, primarily tea, desserts and other foods when looking for a mild lemon flavor. It is very popular in Thai, Chinese and other oriental recipes, which is where most people first encounter it. You may be surprised to find that most of the household cleaning liquids that you use day to day are flavored with lemon grass as opposed to actual lemons! When looking at aromatherapy, lemon grass essential oil is well known for its ability to repel annoying insects such as mosquitoes and fleas.

The history of lemon grass essential oil is quite short compared to many of the other essential oils. There are reports indicating that it was first distilled in the 17th century in the Philippines. It has since become one of the most popular essential oils in India, known locally as 'choomana poolu', which refers to the red grass stems of the plant.

In China, lemon grass is used to treat a myriad of health issues ranging from headaches, to colds and rheumatic pains. In India and Sri Lanka where it is also known as 'fever tea', lemon grass is combined with many other herbs to treat fevers, diarrhea and stomach aches. It is even used in Cuba as a treatment for reducing blood pressure.

The health benefits of using lemon grass essential oil as highlighted above are various and powerful. It can be used to reduce pain and inflammation due to its analgesic properties. Lemon grass essential oil can be used to reduce pain in joints and muscles as well as the various aches caused by viral and bacterial infections such as the flu, fever and various poxes. Its antidepressant properties make it a perfect oil to experience first thing in the morning. It will help you feel energized, motivated and confident. The ideal way to do this is to administer a drop or two to your morning tea, the perfect wake up tonic! The other important properties of lemon grass essential oil include;

antibacterial, anti-pyretic, antiseptic, carminative, deodorant, fungicidal, insecticidal, nervine and sedative.

The main chemical components of lemongrass oil are myrcene, citronellal, geranyl acetate, nerol, geraniol, neral and traces of limonene and citral.

It is important to be aware that lemon grass essential oil can irritate sensitive skin, so be sure to perform a spot test before applying to your skin. It should also be avoided during pregnancy, and use on children under 12 is not recommended.

Bergamot (*Citrus Bergamia*)

Bergamot is a plant that produces a type of citrus fruit. The essential oil comes from the rind or peel of the fruit. The scent of bergamot essential oil is very similar to other citrus based essential oils. The citrus scent is sweet and fruity with a warm, slightly spicy quality. It is often compared to the smell of neroli and lavender essential oils. The oil has a watery viscosity and is generally green with a slightly yellow tinge. Its desirable, strong aroma makes it a popular flavor in many perfumes. One of its most famous application is in tea, unknown too many 'Earl Grey' tea is created by adding bergamot essential oil to black tea.

Like most other essential oils, bergamot has that interesting little history. The origin of bergamot can be traced to South East Asia, but has since been introduced to Europe where it thrives, particularly in Italy. The name is derived from the Italian city, Bergamo in Lombardy, where the oil was first sold (supposedly by famous explorer Columbus!). It has reportedly been used since the sixteenth century as a remedy for fever and as an antiseptic.

Recent Italian research has confirmed that bergamot essential oil has a wide range of uses in aromatherapy. Ranging from curing skin diseases to fighting mouth and urinary tract infections. Some of the highlights include its ability to relax and soothe. The flavonoids in bergamot essential oil will help soothe nerves, anxiety, stress and reduce nervous tension. This ties in well to two more of its key properties, an anti-depressant and stimulant. Like many of thr essential oils, bergamot is great to use first thing in the morning to feel energetic, strong and joyful. Other important properties of bergamot essential oil include; antibiotic, analgesic, disinfectant, digestive aid, deodorant, febrifuge, anti-spasmodic and antiseptic.

The essential oil is composed of various chemical constituents and includes a-pinene, myrcene, limonene, a-bergaptene, b-bisabolene, linalool, linalyl acetate, nerol, neryl acetate, geraniol, geraniol acetate and a-terpineol.

When looking at safety with bergamot essential oil it is very important to make sure the oil doesn't come into contact with sunlight. One of its components, bergaptene becomes poisonous if exposed to sunlight. Keep the oil stored in a dark bottle in a dark place. The oil also creates photo-sensitivity so you should avoid sunlight if you have applied the essential oil to your skin within the last 24 hours. Aside from this, bergamot essential oil is considered to be relatively non-toxic and non-irritant.

Helichrysum (*Helichrysum italicum*)

Helichrysum essential oil is one of the most powerful oils in production. Unfortunately it doesn't have the popularity it deserves due to its higher price point compared to other essential oils. I'm sure after reading a bit about its properties you'll agree! It is often nicknamed the 'Everlasting' or 'Immortal' essential oil due to its exceptionally long shelf life. It is important to make sure you are purchasing Helichrysum essential oil from the species highlighted above, 'Helichrysum Italicum', as there are over 600 species of Helichrysum and many are not suitable for therapeutic use. The oil has a strong straw-like, fruity smell. There is a honey and tea undertone to the aroma. The color generally ranges between a light yellow and red, with a watery viscosity. The best Helichrysum essential oil comes from Corsica, a small island off the coast of France.

Unlike most essential oils, the historical documentation of helichyrsums use in medicine and cuisine is scant. One of the key historical notes comes from Holmes, stating that the plant has been used in herbal medicine since the time of Ancient Greece. It has also been a well-known and popular traditional medicine in South Africa. They have been using it to treat rheumatism and to keep their energy levels high whilst up in the mountains. They refer to it as 'sewejaartjie' which is derived from the belief that the flower heads last for seven years when kept in a jar. Lending further claim to the 'Immortal' nickname! When looking at aromatherapy specifically, however, it is almost impossible to find a reference to Helichrysum essential oil in manuals and catalogs written prior to the early 1980's.

For those familiar with herbal medicine, Helichrysum essential oil is to aromatherapy as Arnica is to Herbalism. Helichrysum is a must have for minor traumas, swelling and scars. It has been studied in Europe for the past few decades, looking at its healing abilities on many skin conditions, nerve regeneration, scar reduction and inflammation of the skin. In France it is marketed heavily as an anti-aging miracle, often referred to as the fountain of youth.

As mentioned above, the health benefits of Helichrysum essential oil are simply outstanding. Its wide range of therapeutic properties include; anti-allergenic, anti-inflammatory, antispasmodic, astringent, diuretic, analgesic, expectorant, cytophylactic, cholagogue and nervine. Its nervine property means that it keeps your immune system in good shape, strengthening and protecting it from disorders. This property, with regular use can aid greatly in anti-aging efforts. Further to this, its cytophylactic property promotes cell health whilst encouraging the production of new cells. This helps in the overall health and growth of the body, justifying the French nickname as the fountain of youth.

The main chemical components of helichrysum oil are a-pinene, camphene, b-pinene, myrcene, limonene, 1,8-cineole, linalool, neryl acetate, nerol, geraniol, eugenol and other b-diketones.

On the note of safety, Helichrysum essential oil is non-toxic, non-sensitizing and non-irritant. It should however, not be used on children under the age of 12, and as always, be sure to perform a spot check before full application to your skin.

Vetiver (Vetiveria zizanioides)

Vetiver is one of those little known essential oils that has a powerful range of therapeutic abilities and a rich, interesting history. The oil has an earthy, almost musty smell. I would liken it to the smell of a damp forest floor. It is amber in color. Vetiver has an amazing effect on both your physical and mental health. It is great at calming anger, irritability and hysteria. Whilst also being able to reduce the appearance of stretch marks and wrinkles. Vetiver essential oil is commonly referred to as the oil of tranquility due to its calming effects.

Vetiver has a long and rich history dating back to the 12th century. In India it has been used to make blinds, necessary to keep out the intense heat. When the blinds are sprinkled with water they emit the vetiver scent. This is the country that the nickname 'oil of tranquility' comes from. In Java, the root has been used for centuries in weaving mats and thatching huts. The Vetiver root is used in folk magic for its purported ability to provide safety and increase financial resources. A ritual designed to promote personal safety calls for inhaling Vetiver while visualizing one's body as being sealed off from negative energies. The Ancient Chinese had a belief that vetiver essential oil had high calmative power, which could cool the system, energize brain cells, bring stability to emotions and invigorate dry skin. They also used the oil to treat Yin deficiency, which is effectively depression. In the Middle Ages it was sought after for its popular scent, along with Lime and Rosewood essential oils.

The health benefits of Vetiver Essential Oil can be attributed to its properties as an anti-inflammatory, antiseptic, aphrodisiac, cicatrisant, nervine, sedative, tonic and vulnerary substance. The oils soothing and cooling anti-inflammatory effects are particularly good at providing relief from inflammation in both the circulatory and nervous system. It can also be used to treat the inflammation caused by sun stroke, sun burns and dehydration. As an antiseptic, it has found much popularity in countries such as India, where the conditions provide bacteria with optimal conditions for growth. The essential oil is great at stopping the growth of Staphylococcus Aureus, the bacteria that is responsible for causing sepsis. This is a very safe essential oil, meaning it can be used directly on wounds or taken internally to prevent infection.

On the other side of its therapeutic effects, vetiver is regarded as a great aphrodisiac. When a few drops are added to a beverage it can enhance libido and arouses feelings of sexual desire!

The main chemical components of vetiver essential oil are benzoic acid, vetiverol, furfurol, a and b-vetivone, vetivene and vetivenyl vetivenate.

When looking at safety precautions, Vetiver essential oil comes with very few. It is non-sensitizing, non-irritant and non-toxic. The only precaution I recommend is to perform the standard spot test before applying this oil to your skin. As always, exercise extreme caution when using on children and pregnant women.

Sweet Orange (*Citrus sinensis*)

Orange is one of my favorite essential oils for promoting happiness and warmth. It has a wonderfully sweet, fresh and tangy smell. The color of the oil ranges from yellow to orange and is watery in viscosity. It has a shelf life of roughly half a year. The essential oil is extracted by cold-pressing the orange peel. Next time you peel an orange or another citrus fruit, try squeezing a part of the rind between your fingers and you should be able to smell the intense aroma of the essential oil. It is great to have on hand to deal with colds and flu, stimulating the lymphatic system and supporting the foundation of collagen in your skin.

The name of the orange fruit is presumed to be derived from the Sanskrit 'Narangah'. After being translated through various languages it arrived finally at the English name, orange. The orange plant is believed to be native to South East Asia, with records dating back over 7000 years. A common agreement amongst historians is that oranges were first grown in orchards by the Chinese around the time of the 1st century. The nobles of the time became very fond of the fruit and its delicious fragrance which lead the growers to cultivating larger and tastier oranges to please them. In Europe, records indicate that the Roman Empire first encountered oranges in the 1st century BC. Persian traders were responsible for this introduction. Finally, it was introduced to America by Spanish conquistadors. Today, Brazil is by far the leading producer of oranges in the world, accounting for more than half of the world's total production! The actual essential oil however is primarily produced in France, Italy and Israel.

The impressive therapeutic properties of orange oil are antiseptic, anti-depressant, antispasmodic, anti-inflammatory, carminative, diuretic, cholagogue, sedative and tonic. With this wide versatility and the affordability of orange essential oil, it is one of the most popular in aromatherapy. Its anti-depressant property is perfect for bringing cheer and happiness to a room. It is another one of those oils I choose to experience early in the morning, to bring a sense of well-being and energy to my day. You can simply add a drop to a meal or drink, or diffuse it for that emotional lift. As a carminative, the oil helps remove excess gas from the intestines and digestive system. This is a common and often overlooked health concern. When gas forms in the intestines and pushes upwards it can cause chest pains, indigestion and general discomfort. Orange essential oil helps prevent this by relaxing our abdominal muscles, allowing the gas to escape.

The main chemical components of orange essential oil are a-pinene, sabinene, myrcene, limonene, linalool, citronellal, neral and geranial. With 85-95% of the oil consisting of limonene, a strong antioxidant.

There are a couple of safety concerns to be aware of when looking at orange essential oil. Do not use the oil on children under the age of 6. It is mildly photosensitive so you should avoid direct sunlight for up to 12 hours after use. It is very important to do spot tests before applying this essential oil fully as it has been known to cause sensitization in some cases. Finally, it is not recommended to use this essential oil when pregnant.

Myrrh (*Commiphora myrrha*)

Myrrh essential oil is pale yellow to amber in color. It has a warm, slightly musty smell. It comes from a small tree that will grow up to roughly 5 meters in height with light bark and twisted branches. The tree has just a few leaves and small white flowers. The essential oil is extracted by steam distillation of the oleoresin-gum.

Myrrh has one of the richest histories of all the essential oils, which may come as no surprise if you are familiar with the Christian Bible. The fragrant aroma has been the inspiration of merchants, priests, aristocrats and poets for many thousands of years. It has been held in an esteemed position in many civilizations over the course of history, due to its effectiveness as a medicinal herb. The name, myrrh, is thought to come from the Arabic word 'morr' which translates to bitter. Ancient historian Herodotus recorded that the Egyptians used myrrh as an embalming agent, as well as burning it to rid their houses of fleas and mosquitoes. It was also popularly used as a mask to hide the stench that lingered due to a lack of good hygiene and sanitary standards.

Famously, during the time of Christ, myrrh was given by the wise men as one of the three gifts. Alongside frankincense and gold. Myrrh was one the most highly valued commodities during this time and was cherished as a precious oil. The Hebrew people used it to anoint the altar and other sacred vessels in the Jewish Temples. Another famous use of the time was in the purification process that women used to beautify themselves before being presented to King Ahasurerus of the Medes when he was choosing a queen.

Myrrh was also a big part of Indian Ayurvedic medicine. They used it treat a myriad of health conditions ranging from mouth ulcers to gingivitis to respiratory conditions. At around the middle of the seventh century AD, myrrh was introduced to both Tibetan and Chinese medicines. The Chinese call myrrh 'mo yao' and have used it since the time of the Tang Dynasty as a wound healer.

In the 1700's famous herbalist Samuel Thomson named myrrh as one of the most essential herbs for improving health, much to the anger of doctors at the time! He was most fond of myrrh's antiseptic and cleansing properties. Myrrh has maintained its place as a staple in aromatherapy and herbalism right up to the modern age.

Myrrh has an impressive list of therapeutic properties; anti-catarrhal, anti-inflammatory, antimicrobial, antiphlogistic, antiseptic, astringent, balsamic, carminative, cicatrisant, emmenagogue, expectorant, fungicidal, sedative, digestive and pulmonary stimulant, stomachic, tonic, uterine and vulnerary.

Some of the key uses, taking into account these properties include applying the essential oil to a burner or vaporizer in order to treat bronchitis, catarrh, coughs and colds. It is also a fantastic scent to have in the air whilst meditating or simply relaxing. As the Ayurvedics found out thousands of years ago, it is a great oil to add to a mouthwash in order to treat ulcers and other dental infections, taking full advantage of its antimicrobial property. As a tonic, myrrh essential oil contributes to the strengthening and improvement of all the bodies systems and organs. It protects them from bacterial infections, viruses and premature aging.

When considering safety whilst using myrrh essential oil it is important to point out that pregnant women should never use it. It stimulates the uterus and could therefore result in a miscarriage. As with all essential oils be sure to exercise extreme care when using the on or around children, always check with your doctor before use.

Random fact – Myrrh is referred to 156 times in the Bible, more than any other oil!

Cinnamon, Leaf (Cinnamomum verum)

Cinnamon essential oil is another oil with a rich and fascinating history. It possesses a spicy, warm and musky smell and the color generally ranges from yellow to red-brown. The viscosity is slightly thicker than water. Cinnamon is a popular essential oil in aromatherapy. It has very powerful anti-rheumatic properties and is a great aid in fighting coughs and colds.

True cinnamon is native to Sri Lanka and the south east coast of India. Despite this exotic, distant origin, cinnamon was widely known and popular throughout the ancient world. It is believed that the Arabs first introduced the spice to the west and controlled the trade for centuries via their extensive trading routes. It is here that we may learn that exaggerated stories began use as marketing techniques, thanks to this quote from Herodotus.

"Their manner of collecting the Cinnamon is still more extraordinary. In what particular spot it is produced they themselves are unable to certify. There are some who assert that it grows in the region where Bacchus was educated and their mode of reasoning is by no means improbable. These affirm that the vegetable substance which we, as instructed by the Phoenicians, call Cinnamon, is by certain large birds carried to their nests constructed of clay, and placed in the cavities of inaccessible rocks. To procure it thence, the Arabians have contrived this stratagem: - they cut in very large pieces the dead bodies of oxen, asses or other beasts of burden and carry them near these nests: they then retire to some distance; the birds soon fly to the spot and carry these pieces of flesh to their nests, which not being able to support the weight, fall in pieces to the ground. The Arabians take this opportunity of gathering the Cinnamon which they afterwards dispose of to different countries." – Herodotus, ancient historian.

This and other such stories were circulated to prevent the true origin of cinnamon from becoming common knowledge. This prevented competition and kept the price high! Up until around 1500 AD the Arabs controlled the trade of Cinnamon and spread it worldwide. It is believed that the name comes from the Greek word 'Kinnamom' which means tube or pipe. The Greeks primarily used the oil for temple incense whilst the Egyptians used it for foot massages as well as curing digestive pains. They also used it as an ingredient in mulled wines, sedatives and love potions.

The wide range of cinnamon essential oils therapeutic properties include; antiseptic, antibiotic, antispasmodic, aphrodisiac, astringent, cardiac, carminative, emmenagogue, insecticide, stimulant, stomachic, tonic and vermifuge.

Cinnamon essential oil is a natural pain reliever. You can use it to soothe pain in your muscles, aches, joint stiffness and chronic pain. Regularly massaging with cinnamon essential oil will reduce inflammation long term. The aroma of cinnamon essential oil is uplifting and warm. It is an easy way to lift your mood and make you feel at ease. It is as simple as inhaling from your vial of cinnamon oil for a minute to get this uplifting effect. Due to the high amount of eugenol in cinnamon essential oil, which is also the main constituent of clove essential oil it can provide instant relief from tooth aches and pain. If you do not have clove oil to hand, cinnamon is a great alternative.

The main chemical components of the essential oil, obtained from the leaves, are eugenol, eugenol acetate, cinnamic aldehyde and benzyl benzoate

It is important to ensure that your oil is extracted from the leaf and not from the bark as the leaf oil is non-toxic. That isn't to say it is completely safe. Caution must be exercised when inhaling the oil, as it can cause irritation to the mucus membranes. The oil is an emmenagogue and so should never be used by a pregnant woman. Finally, be sure to not use the oil on children under six years old, and to provide extra dilution when using it on children between the ages of six and twelve. As with every essential oil, ensure a spot test is carried out before using it for the first time.

Clary Sage (Salvia sclarea)

Whilst not a cheap essential oil, clary sage comes with a host of health benefits. Ranging from easing depression and anxiety to relieving congested complexions. The oil is a pale yellow and possesses a sweet and nutty fragrance. It has a watery viscosity. Clary sage essential oil is extracted by steam distillation of the flowering tops and leaves.

Clary sage has a brief but interesting history that reveals itself in the names which were given to the plant. Medieval authors called the herb 'clear eye' as it was considered to be beneficial when dealing with visual problems. 'Clary' is derived from the Latin word 'clarus' which means clear. A well-known herbalist from these times, known as Nicholas Culpepper was at the forefront of using the plants seeds in vision healing. During the Middle Ages, clary sage was known as 'Oculus Christi', otherwise known as the eyes of Christ. Over in Germany it was called 'Muscatel Sage', due to its resemblance to muscatel wine. Dishonest merchants of the time would adulterate their muscatel wine with clary sage. This often produced a heightened sense of intoxication and disorientation. The name was derived from the combination of these two products.

As you may expect from an essential oil, the therapeutic properties of clary sage are just as varied and powerful as the rest. The major therapeutic properties of clary sage essential oil include; antidepressant, antiphlogistic, anti-spasmodic, aphrodisiac, deodorant, emmenagogue, hypotensive, nervine, sedative, tonic and uterine.

As pointed to previously, clary sage essential oil will improve eyesight and protect your eyesight from aging. It is used in many eye cleansers and eye drops. This, as you can see from the large list of therapeutic properties above is not where the health benefits stop! The oil is very useful in treating spasms and related ailments such as headaches, coughs, muscle cramps and spasmodic cholera. It causes the nerve impulses to relax and prevents the uncontrollable spasms from occurring. Often associated with the euphoric nature of clary sage, the oil is often used as an aphrodisiac. It can provide a great boost to libido and sexual desire and studies have shown it to be equally effective in males and females.

The chief components of clary sage essential oil are Sclareol, Alpha Terpineol, Geraniol, Linalyl Acetate, Linalool, Caryophyllene, Neryl Acetate and Germacrene-D. The oil is fairly unusual due to the fact it is composed more from esters than other substances.

Clary sage is generally a safe essential oil, but there are naturally a few safety precautions that must be adhered to. Clary sage is not safe to use during the first trimester of pregnancy. It is not recommended that you combine clary sage essential oil with alcohol as it will produce a stronger sense of intoxication. Finally, inhalation of clary sage should be in small amounts to prevent excessive states of euphoria! Be sure to perform a spot test before applying this essential oil to your skin, as always.

Cypress (Cypressus sempervirens)

Cypress is a less common essential oil, however the clear, fresh smell is a great experience when you are feeling agitated, stressed or angry. It is most often used for improving circulation and sorting out coughs and bronchitis. The oil has a watery viscosity and is almost colorless with a very weak tinge of yellow. It has a lightly spicy, woody, somewhat masculine aroma.

Cypress is an evergreen tree with deep green foliage, small flowers and round brown cones with seed nuts inside. The tree's wood is very hard and durable and is a light red color. Due to the strength of the wood it was used to make sarcophagi for Ancient Egyptian mummies and the Greeks often used it to make statues of their many gods. This led to the belief that cypress held powerful protective forces and symbolized life after death. This symbolic longevity was continued by the ancient Greeks and Romans through the use of the word 'sempervirens', which you may notice is in its botanical name above. It means ever-living.

The therapeutic properties of cypress oil are astringent, antiseptic, antispasmodic, deodorant, diuretic, haemostatic, hepatic, styptic, sudorific, vasoconstrictor, respiratory, tonic and sedative. These properties are what gives cypress essential oil its soothing, calming effect on a stressed or irritated person. Its use as a vasoconstrictor can have a valuable effect on hemorrhoids and varicose veins. It is a very helpful oil to have on hand in the case of excess fluids, for examples; bleeding, nose bleeds, bronchitis, heavy menstruation and heavy perspiration. The antispasmodic property can be a great aid when suffering from asthma, influenza and emphysema.

The main components of cypress oil are a-pinene, camphene, sabinene, b-pinene, d-3carene, myrcene, a-terpinene, terpinolene, linalool, bornyl acetate, cedrol and cadinene.

When looking at safety precautions for cypress essential oil it is considered non-toxic, non-irritant and non-sensitizing. However, it should not be used on pregnant women or children under the age of six. As always please carry out a spot test before applying fully to your skin.

Sweet Basil (Ocimum basilicum)

Basil essential oil has a watery viscosity and is pale green of color, with a subtle yellow tinge. The scent is light, clear and peppery. This crisp smelling essential oil is very common in aromatherapy practice due to its ability to awaken the mind to clarity of thought. It is great at calming anxiety and nerves whilst also being able to ease menstrual pains, reduce sinus congestion and relieve the symptoms of fever. It is one of the first essential oils I turn to when suffering from a cold. It is extracted via steam distillation from the flowering tops and leaves.

Basil originates from the Pacific Islands and tropical Asia but is now cultivated throughout the world. Basilicum comes from the Greek word 'Basilicos' meaning 'king' or 'royal'. A very popular herb in India, it is held sacred to Krishna and Vishnu and the leaves of the herb are often chewed before taking part in religious ceremonies. Due to its supposed protective qualities, a basil leaf is placed on the chest of a Hindu when resting. It also has a large history of use in Ayurvedic and Chinese medicine.

The wide range of basil essential oils impressive therapeutic qualities include; analgesic, antidepressant, antispasmodic, anti-venomous, carminative, cephalic, diaphoretic, digestive, emmenagogue, expectorant, febrifuge, insecticide, nervine, stomachic, sudorific, tonic and stimulant. These properties give basil oil a refreshing effect when inhaled or consumed, so it is commonly used for treating nervous tension, mental fatigue, migraines and depression. As an analgesic its ability to soothe aches and pains makes it a top choice for treating arthritis, burns, muscular soreness, bruises, scars and headaches. A further top use of basil essential oil that I love to employ is its ability to reduce the symptoms of nausea. This is particularly helpful when suffering from motion sickness.

Basil oil has various chemical compounds that include a-pinene, camphene, b-pinene, myrcene, limonene, cis-ocimene, camphor, linalool, methyl chavicol, y-terpineol, citronellol, geraniol, methyl cinnamate and eugenol.

There are a couple of safety precautions to be aware of when it comes to basil essential oil. You should not use this oil if you are pregnant and it should not be used on children under the age of six. I recommend using basil only in very small amounts as high doses might have a carcinogenic effect. Especially in basil oils that have a high quantity of methyl chavicol. Finally be sure to avoid this oil if you are suffering from a liver condition.

A quick note on proprietary blends

Proprietary blends of essential oils are specially formulated 'recipes' which are combinations of a mixture of different essential oils. These can be great for newcomers to essential oils as they often have specific applications as remedies for particular conditions. However, I find that once you have gained some practical knowledge regarding the therapeutic use of essential oils it is often better to purchase single oils for two reasons. One, because with a number of different single oils you can make your own special blends for specific treatments (a few of which will be suggested later in this book); and two, because it is often more economical to do so. You should ensure that, as with any essential oil purchases, blends are purchased only from reputable dealers.

Although the above list is not exhaustive, it is a good basis for starting out in the world of essential oils. With these forming the fundamentals of your collection, it will be possible to treat all manner of symptoms and conditions due to their sheer versatility.

Chapter 3 – Introduction to Carrier Oils

What are carrier oils?

Carrier oils are highly important substances in the world of essential oils. These allow us to sufficiently dilute essential oils for their safe therapeutic use, and often have special therapeutic properties themselves. Carrier oils are typically plant based, and are derived from the nut, seed or kernel of a plant. They are normally high in fatty acids, as well as vitamins, minerals and nutrients. And because of their typically neutral characteristics, carrier oils are perfect for use with active, volatile ingredients such as essential oils. Unlike essential oils, carrier oils generally have fewer restrictions on their safe usage due to their more neutral characteristics.

Why do we need to use carrier oils?

As the pure aromatic essence of organic materials, essential oils contain some volatile and highly concentrated natural compounds. It is thanks to these volatile compounds that we can harness essential oils for some impressive therapeutic applications; however, these same volatile compounds can cause severe irritation to the skin, if applied undiluted. While a few essential oils can be administered 'neat', it is generally always recommended to use a carrier oil when taking essential oils for therapeutic purposes.

How are carrier oils different to essential oils?

As discussed briefly earlier, essential oils are *not really oils*. They are in fact *lipophilic* solutions. This term describes substances that are attracted to fats or lipids. Typically, solutions which are lipophilic are also water repellant, and vice versa. Think for example of the interaction between oil and water; this is what would occur if you attempted to combine an essential oil with a water based carrier instead of an oil based one. Additionally, when kept for a long time, essential oils do not spoil or go rancid, but lose their potency through oxidation (chemical reaction with the air). It is similar, for example, to what happens to spices used for food when left secreted away in a cupboard for a long period of time. These do not go bad *per se*, but instead lose their flavor and potency over time. On the other hand, carrier oils can go rancid if stored for a long period of time due to their high fat content.

Despite their differences, however, essential oils and carrier oils share several complementary qualities that make them work well together when used therapeutically. Firstly, both essential oils and carrier oils typically have their own positive therapeutic effects – for example, when combined together in an aromatherapy treatment, an essential oil might account for the antiviral or antiseptic properties of a mixture, while the same solution's carrier oil can be the source of its nourishing vitamins. Secondly, both essential oils and carrier oils are normally easily absorbed into the skin, allowing them to enter the bloodstream relatively quickly. This is important if the full therapeutic effects of essential oils are to be enjoyed, and is also why mineral oils (such as 'baby oil') cannot be used as carriers. These are typically comprised of larger molecules that are difficult for the skin to absorb (which, given the fact that these are normally derived from petrochemicals, is indeed a good thing!). Third, the chemically inert nature of carrier oils makes them perfect for use with more volatile essential oils. This means that the natural properties of essential oils that are so important for their therapeutic use are not diminished or altered when combined with carrier oils.

Does the aroma of carrier oils interfere with or change the aroma of essential oils?

Generally speaking, the aroma of an essential oil will not be affected by the aroma of a carrier oil. The latter generally have a neutral to faintly sweet smell, which is overpowered by the strong scent that is typical of an essential oil. If you do notice that a carrier oil has a strong smell, it may be due to the fact that it has gone rancid. This is indicated by an astringent, bitter odor. If you believe that a carrier oil has gone rancid, it should be discarded. Additionally, because carrier oils can have a fairly neutral aroma, it is important to store them in glass to prevent unwanted odors being imparted in them from other materials (such as some plastics).

Things to look for when buying carrier oils

As when buying essential oils, the quality of carrier oils is very important – especially when being used therapeutically. The best quality carrier oils for therapeutic use are typically cold pressed. These are sometimes available in supermarkets for basic carriers (such as grapeseed oil); however, care should be taken to check the label that the product has indeed been produced through this process. This is indicated by the use of either the term 'cold pressed' or 'cold expeller pressed'. If there is no extraction method listed on the label, it is safe to presume that the product has not been cold pressed. Heat and solvent extraction (which are the standard methods of obtain plant oils, aside from cold pressing) can damage some of the delicate compounds and nutrients in carrier oils.

Blending carrier oils with essential oils

Before blending carrier oils with essential oils, it is important to take into consideration a few key factors to create an appropriate blend. The first and most obvious consideration is the ratio of the mixture – that is what percentage of the blend will be comprised of essential oil(s) and what percentage will be carrier oil. Typically, carrier oils constitute the lion's share of the mixture, but it is important to make sure the concentration is neither too diluted, nor too potent. To avoid these problems, follow recipes for blending essential oils and carrier oils, and always patch test a mixture on a small area of skin to test for irritation before beginning a full treatment. Second, it is important to choose carrier oils that are complementary to the essential oils being used, and the overall treatment for which the blend will be applied. For example, when creating a mixture for use as a topical skin treatment, you should include a carrier oil with properties that are good for skin treatment, such as avocado oil. These factors will be discussed later in greater detail when we cover the top 10 carrier oils for use in aromatherapy.

Storing carrier oils

Carrier oils should be stored in similar conditions to essential oils. Neither carrier oils nor essential oils like being exposed to extreme or sudden heat, and dark glass containers are best to extend their shelf life. Because all carrier oils have different properties, there is no set time period for how long they should last. One kind of oil may last for decades, while another type could go rancid within a year. The shelf life of some carrier oils will be discussed in more detail further below when we take a look at the top 10 carrier oils.

Chapter 4 – The Top 10 Carrier Oils

With the basics of carrier oils covered above, I will now turn to an examination of the top 10 carrier oils for use with essential oils. These are some of the most used and useful carrier oils in aromatherapy. Like essential oils, carrier oils have their own distinct properties that should be considered when being selected for therapeutic usage with essential oils. Some carrier/essential oils make particularly good combinations, thanks to their complementary properties. The following is a list of the top 10 essential oils, their various qualities, and the types of treatments they are best used with.

Avocado Oil

Avocado (*Persea Americana*) is a highly viscous carrier oil derived from the fleshy pulp surrounding the seed of the avocado. Unadulterated, the oil has a nutty flavor, is very high in monounsaturated fatty acids, and is edible. When extracted through cold pressing, avocado oil is a vibrant emerald green. It is also a very viscous oil, is rich in vitamin A and D, and also contains significant amounts of lecithin (good for dry skin, eczema, stress and anxiety), potassium, and vitamin E. Because of these qualities, it is often a good choice when combined with essential oils for skin treatments. Typically, because of its viscosity and expensiveness, it is often blended with cheaper carrier oils at ratio of about 10 to 30 percent avocado oil. Avocado oil has a shelf life of about 12 months.

Borage Seed Oil

Borage oil is obtained from the seed of the borage plant (*Borago officinalis*), an annual herb native to the Mediterranean. This plant is also known by its common name, 'starflower'. Borage oil contains high concentrations of *y-linolenic acid*, which lends it both anti-inflammatory and anti-thrombotic qualities. As such, it is useful in treatments of rheumatological conditions, such as arthritis or gout, and in the prevention of the occurrence of clotting disorders, such as deep-vein thrombosis. Borage oil is also a good choice when treating skin conditions, such as acne. As it is a very expensive oil, borage can be blended with other carriers while still retaining its unique therapeutic qualities. The shelf life of borage oil is around 9-12 months.

(N.B. people with liver conditions should avoid borage oil as it contains compounds which may be hepatotoxic. Additionally, borage oil should be avoided while pregnant as some studies have indicated that it may have the effect of inducing early labor.)

Coconut Oil

Lightly textured, clear and odorless, fractionated coconut (*Cocos nicifera*) oil is derived from the inner nut of the fruit (or nut) of the coconut palm. It bears many distinct therapeutic properties, including antibiotic, germicidal, antiviral and antifungal qualities. It can be used either on its own or in combination with other more expensive carrier oils. It is also relatively inexpensive and has an indefinite shelf life, making it a great carrier oil to keep on hand.

Evening Primrose Oil

This extremely fine textured and lightly scented oil is derived from the seeds of the Evening Primrose herbaceous flower (*Oenothera biennis*), native to the Americas. Like borage oil, evening primrose contains high amounts of the anti-inflammatory and anti-thrombotic y-linoleic acid, and is rich in other omega-6 fatty acids. One of the most expensive carrier oils available, it is usually diluted with a more inexpensive oil such as grapeseed, at a ratio of as little as 10 percent evening primrose. The shelf life of evening primrose is rather short at around six months, and can be extended with the addition of a small amount of a long life oil, such as wheatgerm.

Grapeseed Oil

Grapeseed oil is a very useful commodity in aromatherapy because of its inexpensiveness and versatility. As the name suggests, it is derived from the seed of the grape, and is a very thin, clear oil with a sweet, slightly nutty aroma. Various varietals of the common grape (*Vitus vinifera*) may be used in its production, with Chardonnay and Riesling being two examples. Thanks to its versatility, grapeseed oil can be used in a number of applications, from massage to skin treatments. High in linoleic acid (distinct from y-linoleic acid described earlier), grapeseed has good regenerative and moisturizing properties for the skin. Due to being an abundant byproduct of the wine making process, grapeseed oil is typically very inexpensive. One of the major downsides of grapeseed oil, however, is its short shelf life of 6-12 months.

Macadamia Nut Oil

Derived from the pressed nuts of the macadamia tree *(Macadamia Integrifolia)*, macadamia nut oil is another very useful therapeutic carrier oil. High in the omega-9 fatty acid, *oleic acid*, macadamia oil has useful anti-inflammatory properties. It also contains the highest levels of *palmitoleic acid* of any nut; this acid is found in the skin oil, *sebum*, which is found in higher quantities in younger skin. Therefore, it can be good for improving skin elasticity and reducing dryness. Macadamia oil is sometimes referred to as a 'vanishing oil' as it is absorbed quickly into the skin, thanks to its fine composition. Because of its excellent cosmetic properties, macadamia oil is a good choice for use with aromatherapy treatments aimed at reducing the appearance of scars or blemishes. The shelf life of macadamia oil is about 12 months.

Pomegranate Seed Oil

As the name suggests, this oil is derived from the pressed seed of the fruit of the pomegranate tree (*Punica granatum*). This carrier oil is particularly high in antioxidants (such as polyphenol), which are not only very beneficial for skin regeneration, but are also may be useful for fighting heart disease, general aging and some cancers. It also contains concentrations of *punic acid* which has a great effect in reducing inflammation and swelling. High levels of vitamin E in pomegranate oil are also great for the skin. The shelf life of pomegranate oil is around six months.

Sweet Almond Oil

This oil is obtained through a pressing of the dried kernels of the almond tree (*Prunus amygdalus*). Rich in vitamins A, B and E, almond oil is easily absorbed and is great for all skin types. Due to its neutral characteristics, it is an excellent 'basic' carrier oil, and combines well for all therapeutic treatments. Sweet almond oil is relatively inexpensive and can last for up to a year.

Watermelon Seed Oil

A very light oil with a faint aroma, watermelon seed oil is well absorbed by the skin. Due to these characteristics it makes a good choice as an all-purpose carrier oil. It blends well with thicker oils and, due to its indefinite shelf life, can be added as a preservative to other oils which may spoil more quickly.

Wheatgerm Oil

The 'germ' of the wheat grain comprises a high amount of nutrients and is often discarded during the refining of heavily processed flours. This makes wheatgerm a very suitable candidate as a source for a carrier oil. High levels of vitamin E and fatty acids make this oil very nourishing for the skin. Like watermelon seed oil, one highly useful characteristic of wheatgerm oil is as a preservative for carrier oils with a short shelf life. As a very sticky oil, it is best – in any event – to be mixed with other, lighter oils before therapeutic application.

A note on 'non-oil' carriers

Though not strictly oils, there are some products which can act as great carriers for essential oils. Typically referred to as 'butters', solid vegetable fats (such as cocoa and shea butters) can make great carriers for essential oils. They are also excellent moisturizers and can make an excellent complement to aromatherapy massage treatments. Jojoba is another lipid which doesn't quite fit under the 'oil' label, but still exhibits very suitable properties as a carrier. Though normally referred to as an oil (as it resembles an oil in all but its chemical composition), jojoba is in fact a liquid wax. Compared to many carriers, this attribute gives jojoba a superior shelf life. Finally, gels can also act as great carriers for essential oils, such as aloe vera. These are best used for topical applications which can benefit from the soothing qualities of gels, such as an anti-acne treatment.

Chapter 5 – Advanced massage treatments for applying Essential Oils

As mentioned earlier, the practice through which essential oils and other aromatic materials are administered for therapeutic purposes is known as *aromatherapy*. Aside from the basic material ingredients used to conduct aromatherapy treatments, the methods by which they are delivered can also be incredibly important in effecting a positive physiological response from the subject. The following will examine some of the advanced methods for therapeutically applying essential oils, focusing on specialized massage techniques. This will include the introduction and explanation of some basic massage terms and concepts which are important to grasp for those new to the art of massage.

Why is massage important in aromatherapy?

Massage is an important component of the practice of aromatherapy. It is a great way to increase circulation in the body – both in terms of blood flow and energy. This is important when administering essential oils, as their therapeutic effect is intensified by the regular flow of blood throughout the body, as well as engagement with the brain's limbic system (of which, the importance was discussed earlier). Additionally, massage helps us to relax and center the mind, which is particularly important for aromatherapy treatments that are associated with improving one's mental state.

Basic massage terminology

Before we get into the details of delivering aromatherapy via massage, there are first some basic massage concepts that need to be explained. If you have ever given or received a massage before, you may already be familiar with some of these techniques but not have previously known what they are called or what their purpose is. This section will decode some of this massage terminology in order to help you administer aromatherapy through massage most effectively.

Effleurage is a great warm up technique when beginning any massage. It involves applying firm, even pressure with the palms and moving the hands fluidly all over the target area. This is good for increasing blood flow, a good first step of any massage.

Feathering is a very light touch that is barely perceptible to the recipient of the massage and is often applied with the fingertips. This typically has a very soothing and relaxing effect.

Petrissage involves a targeted kneading of specific muscle groups, and can be performed at a superficial or deep level. This is useful for relieving muscle tension and increasing circulation deep in the muscle tissue.

Vibration is a useful technique for treating sore and tender muscles. This involves tapping the body repeatedly and firmly with the fingertips, and rapidly moving the hands in a circular motion while the fingertips are engaged with the muscle.

Finally, *tapotement* refers to the various 'percussive' techniques used to manipulate body tissues. These include *cupping*, which involves creating an arch-shaped hand and striking the body simultaneously with the heal of the palm and the fingertips; *pummeling*, which employs a loosely made fist to gently but firmly strike to tissue; and *hacking*, which consists of a series of rapid 'karate chop' motions made along the targeted area.

Raindrop technique

There are many different styles of massage which can be complementary to the practice of aromatherapy. Unfortunately, the spatial limitations of the guide preclude discussing these in great detail (however, do be sure to look for our future guides on aromatherapy for more information on these). *(Update: My new* book *"Essential Oil Massage Techniques For Beginners"* has been released and is a direct expansion of this chapter! To find it type this link into your web browser: *http://amzn.to/1C5NDCf*). The following, however, examines a highly popular aromatherapy-based massage technique designed to complement the therapeutic effects of essential oils.

Pioneered by Dr. Gary Young in the 1980s, the *raindrop technique* combines three complementary therapeutic concepts into one holistic treatment: *aromatherapy, the Vita Flex technique,* and *feather stroking.* The raindrop technique is a type of massage therapy which involves stimulating a physiological response from the body through targeting different systems of the body. We are already familiar with the term *aromatherapy*, as the practice of using essential oils for therapeutic purposes. In the case of the raindrop technique, it is in fact the way that the essential oils are applied – in drops along the spine from a height of about six inches – that gives this treatment its name. This sensation has a particularly calmative effect and is good for putting the subject in a relaxed state.

Meanwhile, the *Vita Flex technique* is a therapeutic method which relies on applying pressure to various points on the body to simulate an electric charge in that area. Based on an Ancient Tibetan healing methods, this technique operates on similar principles to the practice of acupuncture, where specific regions or points of the body control or influence different physiological systems. Finally, *feather stroking* refers to the technique of lightly brushing a feather along the length of the spine, forming particular patterns. This shamanic method, native to the Lakota people of North America, is designed to simulate the energy thought to be transmitted by *Aurora Borealis,* or the Northern Lights.

When used together to comprise the 'raindrop technique' the effect of these three distinct elements is a relaxing experience that makes the subject more mentally and physiologically responsive to their aromatherapy treatment.

Massage and safety

This very brief introduction has listed some of the most basic techniques of massage that may be used to complement aromatherapy treatments. It is important at this stage, as with every stage of administering essential oils for therapeutic purposes, to ensure that some safety precautions are highlighted. If the subject has just had surgery performed on the target area, has a communicable disease or fever, or has a history of thrombosis, massage should be avoided. Sensitive areas should also be avoided, such those affected by varicose veins or arthritis, for example. Finally, massage should only be performed on pregnant women on the advice of a doctor.

Chapter 6 – Remedies and Recipes

With all of the 'set-up' of aromatherapy covered, it is useful to have a few basic therapeutic remedies up your sleeve as a beginner. The following chapter will examine some of the most basic but most useful essential oil recipes for treating common complaints and ailments. (*N.B. None of these remedies are a substitute for emergency medical care. If you have suffered a severe injury or acute medical complaint, you should contact your nearest emergency services center. Additionally, if you notice that your condition is not improving or is becoming worse after a few days, you should seek medical treatment.*)

Acne

Acne is an incredibly common complaint that strikes many teenagers or young adults. While the acne can subside over time as hormones settle, it can leave behind unflattering scars and blemishes that can remain visible for life. This aromatherapy treatment helps to clear up acne and reduce the incidence of outbreaks, making the chances of residual scarring less likely.

Ingredients:
- 8 drops of Lavender oil
- 7 drops of Tea Tree oil
- 2 drops of Juniper oil
- 2 drops of Geranium oil
- 2 drops of Chamomile oil
- 30mL of Borage Seed oil *or* Aloe Vera gel

Preparation/Application:
- In a small glass bottle, add carrier oil, followed by each of the essential oils.
- Shake well, until all ingredients are emulsified.
- Apply mixture sparingly to acne affected areas twice daily.
- Continue with treatment for six weeks; if no discernible results

are observed,   increase concentration of Lavender and Tea Tree oils by a few drops each.

Allergies

One of the most frustrating things about coming into nice weather is the simultaneous onset of allergy season. High pollen counts can leave us with runny noses, watery eyes, and itchy, red skin. With the following allergy remedy, you won't have to worry about the beautiful spring weather being ruined by a case of the sniffles again.

Ingredients:
- 3 drops Eucalyptus oil
- 2 drops Rosemary oil
- 2 drops Sandalwood oil
- Blank inhaler

Preparation/Application:
- Apply essential oils to blank inhaler.
- Use inhaler when hay fever/allergy attack strikes.

Appetite Balance

Eating between meals is one of the main reasons for weight gain, bloating and more. However, essential oils can help you balance your appetite so you only need to eat at meal times.

Ingredients:
- 2 drops of Orange oil

Preparation/Application:
- Add to your drinks throughout the day.
- Or inhale from a clean cloth/tissue as desired.

All-Purpose Cleaner

Store bought cleaners may do the job, but it certainly isn't good for your surroundings as it is full of chemicals which results in you inhaling the toxins. A natural essential oil recipe will do a great job and it'll be better for you to be around.

Ingredients:
- 3 drops of Eucalyptus oil
- 2 drops of Rosemary oil

Preparation/Application:
- Fill a spray bottle 3/4 full of water.
- Put the essential oils inside the bottle and use accordingly.

Asthma

Asthma can be a troubling chronic complaint from which many sufferers find few sources of relief. This remedy, applied as a massage oil to avoid irritating the airways, can be used as a regular, ongoing treatment.

Ingredients:
- 6 drops of Lavender oil
- 3 drops of Rosemary oil
- 3 drops of Eucalyptus oil
- 1 drop of Ginger oil
- 15mL of Macadamia Nut oil

Preparation/Application:
- Mix ingredients in a dark glass bottle.
- Shake until combined thoroughly.
- Apply via massage daily to the chest and back.

Anxiety

Essential oils are extremely helpful in stressful circumstances. If you suffer with anxiety this recipe is recommended as it'll calm you down instantly.

Ingredients:
- 2 drops of Rosewood oil
- 1 drop of Roman Chamomile oil
- 1 drop of Sandalwood oil
- 1 tbsp of Avocado oil

Preparation/ Application:
- Mix the essential oils with the carrier oil, keep it in a dark glass bottle and keep it with you throughout the day.
- When you feel tense massage it on the chest for instant relief, or rub it into the insides of your wrists.

Arthritis

Arthritis can be very unpleasant at times. If you need pain relief, look no further.

Ingredients:
- 1 drop of Lavender oil
- 2 drops of Roman Chamomile oil
- 1 drop of Eucalyptus oil
- 1 drop of Peppermint oil
- 1 tbsp of Macadamia Nut oil

Preparation/ Application:
- Dilute the essential oils with the carrier oil.
- Then, gently massage the mixture into those problem areas.

Anti-Bacterial Purposes

Use this recipe to sanitize areas of your body when you come into contact with bacteria. This can be used like a standard anti-bacterial gel on your hands and feet.

Ingredients:
- 2 drops of Tea Tree oil
- 3 drops of Citronella oil
- 1 drop of Lavender oil
- 1 drop of Rosemary oil
- 1 tbsp of Coconut oil

Preparation/ Application:
- Mix the essential oils with the carrier oil and apply to the affected areas.
- This is especially effective when applied to areas of the body with frequent   contact with bacterial hotspots.

Anti-Microbial Purposes

Use this recipe as an effective way to kill microbes around any area of the house.

Ingredients:
- 1 drop of Thyme oil
- 2 drops of Lemongrass oil
- 3 drops of Rosemary oil
- 1 tbsp of Jojoba oil

Preparation/ Application:
- Blend the essential oils well with the jojoba oil and use on surfaces around the house.

Aiding Respiratory Function

Breathe easy with this effective essential oils recipe, it will clear your airway in no time.

Ingredients:
- 1 drop of Ravensare oil
- 2 drops of Eucalyptus oil
- 1 drop of Ponderosa Pine oil
- 1 drop of Myrtle oil
- 1 drop of Cypress oil
- 1 tbsp of Watermelon Seed oil

Preparation/ Application:
- Mix well with the carrier oil and apply through a gentle massage to the chest area.
- This is especially effective if you're experiencing tightness in the chest and have difficulty breathing.

Blood Sugar

Regulate your blood sugar levels with this simple yet effective method using essential oils.

Ingredients:
- 3 drops of Eucalyptus oil
- 1 tbsp of Borage Seed oil

Preparation/Application:
-Mix the two ingredients together in a small bowl
- Massage the mixture into the soles of your feet 1-2 times a day to regulate your blood sugar levels.

Blood Circulation

Get your blood flowing with this simple yet effective recipe.

Ingredients:
- 2 drops of Goldenrod oil
- 1 drop of Cyprus oil
- 3 drops of Marjoram oil
- 1 tbsp of Primrose oil

Preparation/ Application:
- Mix well and apply to various parts of the body. The inside of your wrists is a great spot to massage this blend into your skin. I also recommend the chest, upper back and calves.

Bumps & Burns

Heal burns and bumps quicker with this simple, lavender based recipe. This will soothe as well as naturally disinfect and heal the skin.

Ingredients:
- 4 drops of Lavender oil
- 1 tbsp of Avocado oil

Preparation/ Application:
- Mix well with the carrier oil and apply over any cuts, burns or bumps. If you wish, this can be applied without adding the carrier oil.

Bruises

Naturally heal bruises with essential oils and halve the repair time. This recipe can also relieve pain and soothe the bruise.

Ingredients:
- 1 drop of Yarrow oil
- 1 drop of Sandalwood oil
- 1 drop of Citronella oil
- 1 tbsp of Sweet Almond oil

Preparation/ Application:
- Dilute the essential oils with the almond oil.
- Then, massage into the affected area.

Colds

Dealing with coughs and colds is one of the most common uses for essential oils. This brilliant recipe is sure to have you seeing the better side of your cold in no time at all!

Ingredients:
- 1 drop of Lemongrass oil
- 1 drop of Sandalwood oil
- 2 drops of Tea Tree oil
- 1 tbsp of Primrose oil

Preparation/ Application:
- Mix together and massage into the neck and chest in the same way you would use a proprietary vapor rub.
- As colds are seated primarily in the nose and throat, the diffusion method is the most effective and any of the appropriate essential oils used via a diffuser in the bedroom will alleviate symptoms and tackle the infection.

Congested Chest

This blend is suitable for a congested chest condition possibly due to excess phlegm in the body.

Ingredients:
- 2 drops of Niaouli oil
- 1 drop of Sweet Birch oil
- 1 drop of Lavender oil
- 1 tbsp of Extra Virgin Olive oil

Preparation/ Application:
- Add the essential oils to the olive oil and blend/shake well in a dark glass bottle.
- Then, apply to the chest before bed via a gentle massage. This will help you to breathe easier and get sufficient rest.

Conjunctivitis (Pink Eye) Condition

This is the perfect remedy for relieving redness in the eyes. Conjunctivitis is an infection/condition that affects the eyes. It is often caused by; chlorine, allergens and using dated products on the eyes.

Ingredients:
- 2 drops of Tea Tree oil
- 2 drops of Lavender oil
- 1 tsp of Coconut oil

Preparation/ Application:
- Mix well with any carrier oil to dilute the essential oils.
- Then, carefully apply around both eyes. Try to avoid dripping any of the mixture into the eye. If it comes into contact with the eye, do not wash with water! Instead, rinse the eye with coconut oil or olive oil.

Coughing

To ease an annoying and persistent cough, this recipe is made in the form of a cough elixir. Unlike many normal cough mixtures, this remedy is effective, natural and even tastes great!

Ingredients:
- 1 drop of Peppermint oil
- 1 drop of Eucalyptus oil
- 2 drops of Lemon oil
- 3 tablespoons of Honey

Preparation/Application:
- Mix ingredients together well.
- Take orally every 2-3 hours as needed.

Constipation

Ease the effects of constipation with this effective essential oils method, as it helps to stimulate bowel movement.

Ingredients:
- 1 drop of Ginger oil
- 1 drop of Orange oil
- 1 drop of Rosemary oil
- 1 tbsp of Coconut oil

Preparation/ Application:
- Dilute the essential oils with the carrier oil into a small bowl.
- Massage into your stomach clockwise.

Circulation

Circulation relates to how well blood is able to flow through the body. While the symptoms of poor circulation can seem innocuous (such as coldness of the extremities, and difficulty concentrating) the causes can potentially be more serious (such as arteriosclerosis or diabetes). The following treatment can be highly effective in terms of improving circulation over time.

Ingredients:
- 2 drops of Neroli oil
- 2 drops of Lemon oil
- 2 drops of Cypress oil
- 2 drops of Frankincense oil
- 2 drops of Geranium oil
- 15 mL of carrier oil (Avocado oil works well)

Preparation/Application:
- Combine ingredients together in a small glass bottle.
- Shake well until combined.
- Apply to affected areas via massage.
- Continue treatment as needed.

Croup

Croup is an infection of the voice box and windpipe, most common in children. It is often mild but essential oils can make the infection easier to deal with.

Ingredients:
- 2 drops of Marjoram oil
- 2 drops of Ravensare oil
- 2 drops of Sandalwood oil
- 1 drop of Thyme oil
- 1 tbsp of Avocado oil

Preparation/ Application:
- Dilute the carrier oil with the essential oils and massage onto the chest.
- Consult your health practitioner before applying these essential oils to a young child. They may have an adverse effect.

Calming

When inhaled, eucalyptus oil helps calm tensions and uplifts the spirit, demoting stress whilst promoting relaxation and relief.

Ingredients:
- 25 drops of Eucalyptus oil
- 1 tbsp of Jojoba oil

Preparation/Application:
- Mix the oils together and put into a dark glass bottle.
- Inhale from the bottle as needed.

Chapped Lips

Bring moisture back into your lips with this nourishing formula. It is a much healthier, more natural alternative to the chemical filled lip balm you may already be using.

Ingredients:
- 1 drop of Roman Chamomile oil
- 1 drop of Rosewood oil
- 1 tbsp of Coconut oil

Preparation/ Application:
- Mix together and place in a small tub.
- Apply as many times as you need a day until the issue is gone.

Cellulite

Banish cellulite with this simple yet effective remedy using the natural power of eucalyptus essential oil.

Ingredients:
- 3 drops eucalyptus oil
- 1 tbsp of jojoba oil

Preparation/Application:
- Dry brush the mixture onto the areas that are concerning you, daily.

Cravings

Reduce cravings with essential oils. Calm your taste buds and rein in your appetite using eucalyptus essential oil.

Ingredients:
- 6 drops of eucalyptus oil

Preparation/Application:
- Diffuse the oil into the rooms you spend the most time in.

Detoxification

Detoxify with essential oils and get rid of harmful substances in the body and purify your airways.

Ingredients:
- 3 drops of Juniper oil
- 1 tbsp of Macadamia Nut oil

Preparation/Application:
- Diffuse the mixture in the room you spend the most time in.
- Spend a few hours relaxing whilst taking deep breaths.

Dust Allergy

If you've got a bad allergy to dust, diffuse this blend in your house and your worries should be over.

Ingredients:
- 3 drops Melissa oil
- 1 drop Geranium oil
- 1 drop Basil oil

Preparation/ Application:
- Diffuse the essential oils in the room you spend the most time in or place them in an empty inhaler and take in as much as necessary.

Dermatitis

Dermatitis is a result of eczema and skin inflammation. Essential oils can bring back moisture into the skin and repair the damage quickly and naturally.

Ingredients:
- 3 drops Frankincense oil
- 1 drop Tea Tree oil
- 2 drops Orange oil

Preparation/ Application:
- Mix all the essential oils together with a tablespoon of a carrier oil of your choice. I recommend sweet almond or extra virgin olive oil for this recipe.
- Apply on a clean tissue and rub into the affected areas for a few minutes to relieve irritation.

Dry Skin

Dry skin is a killer in those cold winter months or if you suffer from it generally. Essential oils are a natural way to combat and relieve itchiness that comes from dry skin as well as moisturizing the areas properly.

Ingredients:
- 1 drop of Rosewood oil
- 1 drop of Sandalwood oil
- 1 tbsp of Sweet Almond oil

Preparation/ Application:
- Dilute the essential oils with the almond oil and apply to the dry skin with a light massage.

Earache

If you suffer from the occasional earache and can't do anything to relieve the pain, try this basic essential oil recipe to instantly rid you of discomfort and pain.

Ingredients:
- 2 drops of Sandalwood oil
- 2 drops of Roman Chamomile oil
- 1 tbsp of Jojoba oil

Preparation/ Application:
- Mix all ingredients together and place 2-3 drops in the painful ear 2-3 times a day as needed.

Eyebrow Thickening

Essential oils can enhance the thickness of your hair, particularly the hair that composes your eyebrows. If you are looking for a thicker and fuller brow, this recipe should do the trick.

Ingredients:
- 2 drops of Rose oil
- 1 drop of Lavender oil
- 1 tbsp of Coconut oil

Preparation/ Application:
- Apply the mixture of ingredients onto the brows every night before bed until you see results and be sure to wash off in the morning.

Ear Infection

An ear infection is usually caused by seasonal weather that weakens the immune system or it can be caused by allergens. This powerful blend can help fight the bacteria that may be causing the infection.

Ingredients:
- 2 drops of Peppermint oil
- 1 drop of Lavender oil
- 1 drop of Rose oil
- 1 tbsp of Coconut oil

Preparation/ Application:
- Mix the ingredients well with the coconut oil.
- Rub the mixture around the outside of the ear and down the neck to treat ear infections.

Energy

Are you constantly lacking energy when you need it most and feel like you need an energy boost? This essential oils recipe is sure to do the trick.

Ingredients:
- 3 drops of Eucalyptus oil
- Or, 3 drops of Peppermint oil
- Or, 3 drops of Lemon oil
- 1 tbsp of Avocado oil

Preparation/Application:
- Either diffuse the essential oil first thing in the morning, or at the time when you need an energy boost. Or mix the essential oils with the carrier oil and massage into your chest.

Facial Cleanser Blend One

The vitamins, minerals and other healthy constituents of essential oils can have a great impact on the appearance of your skin. Add these to an equally rich and soothing carrier oil and you're onto a winner.

Ingredients:
-8 drops of Tea Tree oil
-4 drops of Peppermint oil
-2 drops of Lavender oil
-1 tbsp of Aloe Vera Gel

Preparation/application:
- Blend all the ingredients together in a small bowl
- Begin to apply to the face and neck areas, and gently massage the blend into your skin using small circular movements.
- Allow the blend to absorb into your skin for 2 minutes.
- Gently remove all traces of the oils using a soft cloth soaked in hot water.
- Repeat this process twice a day.

Facial Cleanser Blend Two

Ingredients:
-5 drops of Grapefruit Oil
-5 drops of Lavender Oil
-4 drops of Rosemary Oil
-2 tbsp of Raw Honey

Preparation/application:
-Blend all the ingredients together in a small bowl
-Begin to apply to the face and neck areas, and gently massage the blend into your skin using small circular movements.
- Allow the blend to absorb into your skin for 2 minutes.
-Gently remove all traces of the oils using a soft cloth soaked in hot water.
-Repeat this process twice a day.

Facial Mask

Another brilliant option for improving the health and appearance of your face. This vitamin rich facial mask will leave your skin feeling rejuvenated, firm and healthy.

Ingredients:
-4 drops of Tea Tree Oil
-4 drops of Roman Chamomile Oil
-3 drops of Thyme Oil
-3 drops of Frankincense Oil
-1 tbsp of Apple Cider Vinegar
-1 tbsp of Raw Honey

Preparation/application:
-Blend the ingredients in a small bowl and be sure to use the blend immediately after mixing.
-Apply the blend evenly over your face using a brush or your fingers.
-Leave on your skin for 15-20 minutes.
-Wash off with warm water.
-Repeat once a week.

Floor Cleaner

If you are looking for a healthy, chemical free way of effectively cleaning and disinfecting your floor these antibacterial essential oils are perfect for the job.

Ingredients:
- 3 drops of Eucalyptus oil
- 2 drops of Lemongrass oil
- ¼ cup Distilled White Vinegar
- Quart of Water

Preparation/Application:
- Mix 1/4 cup of distilled white vinegar into a quart of water.
- Add the two essential oils.
- You may add other essential oils to this mixture, such as lemon, pine or spearmint depending on the smell you desire. Be sure to experiment!
- Apply to the floor with a mop. Rinse with clean water after a few minutes of application. The essential oils will work to reduce the smell of the vinegar.

Fever

Fever can accompany all manner of illnesses, meaning that having an effective aromatherapy remedy to help break a fever can be very valuable indeed. Although fever is the body's way of naturally fighting disease, fevers that are left unchecked can be dangerous and lead to complications, from seizures to inflammation of the brain. The antiviral qualities of the essential oils contained in the following recipe can also help the body to fight the source of fever.

Ingredients:
- 2 drops of Eucalyptus oil
- 2 drops of Peppermint oil
- 2 drops of Chamomile oil
- 2 drops of Hyssop oil
- 1 drop of Tea Tree oil
- 1 drop of Black Pepper oil
- 15mL Evening Primrose oil

Preparation/Application:
- Combine Evening Primrose oil with essential oils in a dark glass bottle.
- Shake well until combined.
- Massage small amounts of the mixture into the temples, back of neck, and soles of feet.

Flu

Prevention and treatment with essential oils is the way to go. This quick mixture will have you feeling much better in little time.

Ingredients:
- 1 drop of Lemon oil
- 1 drop of Sandalwood oil
- 2 drops of Tea Tree oil
- 1 tbsp of Grapeseed oil

Preparation/Applications:
-Mix these ingredients together and shake well.
-Apply this mix to the sides of your nose and just under your jaw line to quickly get rid of any discomfort this flu is giving you.

Fatigue

External fatigue also reflects on internal fatigue, this recipe is for use on muscular fatigue or bloated areas, which will revitalize and rejuvenate any tiredness.

Ingredients:
- 3 drops of Peppermint oil
- 3 drops of Ginger oil
- 1 tbsp Extra Virgin Olive oil

Preparation/Application:
- Add peppermint and ginger essential oil to the olive oil.
- Massage firmly into the areas of your body that feel most fatigued.
- Another option is to simply inhale the essential oils individually for a quick lift me up.

Glandular Health Issues

Underactive or overactive; this recipe will balance out your hormones to suit any problem you may be experiencing.

Ingredients:
- 1 drop Myrtle oil
- 2 drops Fleabane oil
- 1 drop Sage oil
- 1 drop Geranium oil
- 1 drop Nutmeg oil
- 1 tbsp jojoba oil

Preparation/ Application:
-Mix well with jojoba oil into a roller bottle and apply topically to glands and any other affected areas.

Headache

Let's face it. Headaches are a nightmare! Whether it's a hangover, dehydration or not enough exercise, this recipe will keep them at bay.

Ingredients:
- 3 drops of Peppermint oil
- 3 drops of Ginger oil
- Blank inhaler

Preparation/Application:
- Add Peppermint or Ginger oils to blank inhaler.
- Inhale deeply as required.

Hay Fever

Spring and summer are the months hay fever sufferers dread because that's when the flowers blossom, triggering allergies in those affected. Use this recipe daily to prevent hay fever symptoms from ruining your summer.

Ingredients:
- 3 drops of Peppermint oil
- 3 drops of Frankincense oil
- Blank inhaler

Preparation/Application:
- Add the essential oils to blank inhaler.
- Inhale deeply as required.

Heartache

Heartache could be caused by tightness in the chest or heart palpitations. To prevent this unpleasant feeling from happening; massage these essential oils onto your chest until the area is relieved.

Ingredients:
- 2 drops of Bergamot oil
- 3 drops of Lavender oil
- 1 drop of Tea Tree oil
- 1 tbsp of Primrose oil

Preparation/Application:
- Mix the essential oils together well with the carrier oil.
- Massage into the chest area, as many times as needed.

Heat Rash

Heat rash is caused when skin rubs together while it's damp. Apply this whenever you feel a rash coming on especially if it's a hot day and you're sweating excessively.

Ingredients:
- 3 drops of Neroli oil
- 3 drops of Patchouli oil
- 1 tbsp of Borage oil

Preparation/Application:
- Combine the essential oils with the Borage oil.
- Massage onto the rash.

Indigestion

I'm sure most of us have had indigestion at one point in our lives; when you ate those wedges from domino's pizza a little too quickly, for example! Inhale these essential oils after eating to clear your digestion.

Ingredients:
- 3 drops of Lemongrass oil
- 3 drops of Grapeseed oil
- 1 tbsp of Coconut oil

Preparation/Application:
- Mix the essential oils and put them in a blank container or tub/bottle.
- Inhale deeply as much as needed.

Immune System Booster

We all have bacteria on our bodies called good bacteria; this is necessary to fight bad bacteria but sometimes our immune system needs a little boost. So, these essential oils are the best way to go.

Ingredients:
- 3 drops Mount Savory oil
- 1 drop Lemon oil
- 2 drops Ravensara oil
- 1 drop Cumin oil
- 1 drop Tansy oil
- 1 tbsp olive oil

Preparation/ Application:
- Mix well with olive oil and apply to affected areas.
- This combination of essential oils can help to make you less susceptible to illnesses.

Ingrown Hair

Ingrown hairs are caused by improper shaving or the aftermath of waxing. To prevent ingrown hairs, add these essential oils to your body lotion and scrub it onto the skin to exfoliate. Tea tree oil is a proven antiseptic/healer that will disinfect any area of the skin when applied.

Ingredients:
- 3 drops of Peppermint oil
- 3 drops of Tea Tree oil

Preparation/Application:
- Add Peppermint or tea tree oils to your body wash/lotion. You can use both if you so wish.
- Shake the mixture well and apply topically.

Insect Bites

It's no secret that essential oils have been used to treat insect bites since the Ancient Egyptians and there's a good reason too; it works! This blend will also help to repel any insects that come your way.

Ingredients:
- 2 drops of Ylang Ylang oil
- 3 drops of Cedarwood oil
- 3 drops of Citronella oil
- 1 tbsp of Macadamia Nut oil

Preparation/Application:
- Add the essential oils to one tablespoon of Macadamia Nut oil and mix well.
- Apply to the insect bites to relieve irritation and speed up the natural healing process.

Influenza

With the chills, aches, headaches, fever and congestion that accompany influenza, most of us would do anything we could to avoid it! The following treatment has two applications: one to try and prevent the onset of flu and two to try and alleviate the symptoms.

Ingredients:
- 2 drops of Eucalyptus oil
- 1 drop of Lemon oil
- 1 drop of Lavender oil
- 1 drop of Sandalwood oil
- 500mL boiling water

Preparation/Application:
- Add all oils along with boiling water to a steam basin.
- Place head over steam basin and cover with a towel. Inhale deeply.
- Repeat treatment twice daily when the symptoms of flu begin to appear.
- The same combination of oils can be added to a bath.

Insomnia

Those of us who experience difficulty sleeping can turn to the power of essential oils to help calm our minds. As in tea form, we can turn to the relaxing properties of chamomile to help us relax before bed. The following recipe is for a massage oil, but the same can just as easily be applied to a diffuser or a hot pre-bedtime bath (leaving out the carrier oil).

Ingredients:
- 10 drops of Roman Chamomile oil
- 5 drops of Lavender oil
- 3 drops of Patchouli oil
- 2 drops of Cedarwood oil
- 30mL of Sweet Almond oil

Preparation/Application:
- Combine ingredients in a dark glass bottle.
- Shake well, ensuring a thorough mixing of ingredients.
- Massage mixture thoroughly into skin, up to one hour before bed.

Intestinal Ailments

Intestinal problems can occur when you're not getting enough fiber or potassium and therefore the intestines get clogged, making them uneasy and uncomfortable for you. To relieve this, use the recipe below.

Ingredients:
- 1 drop Peppermint oil
- 1 drop Chamomile oil
- 2 drops Rosemary oil
- 1 drop Clove oil
- 5 ml vegetable carrier oil

Preparation/ Application:
-Mix the essential oils well to dilute them within the carrier oil.
-This can then be applied to the belly over the area of discomfort.

Itchiness

Itchiness whether it's caused by a rash or an insect can be absolute nightmare. Our natural instinct is to scratch it but we all know that often just makes it worse! Instead apply this emulsion to create a barrier to heal and soothe the skin.

Ingredients:
- 3 drops of Geranium oil
- 2 drops of Agrimony oil
- 1 tbsp of Sweet Almond oil

Preparation/Application:
- Add Geranium and Agrimony oils to one tablespoon of sweet almond oil and mix well.
- Apply onto areas where you are experiencing itchiness.

Joint Pain

Essential oils are a suitable remedy for easing the joints after a long day on your feet or exercising.

Ingredients:
- 2 drops of Wintergreen oil
- 3 drops of Ginger oil
- 1 tbsp of Avocado oil

Preparation/Application:
- Add the essential oils to one tablespoon of avocado oil and mix well.
- Apply to achy joints.

Jet Lag

With long distance travel now the norm rather than the exception, many of us have experienced the unwelcome feeling of jet lag after a long flight. Especially when travelling for business, it can be sometimes impossible to factor in the downtime needed for our bodies to catch up with a new time zone. The following recipe can help to alleviate many of the symptoms associated with jet lag, and can even act as a general 'pick me up' when energy levels are low. As it is administered with an inhaler, this remedy can be made before travelling and conveniently packed in your luggage for use on arrival.

Ingredients:
- 2 drops of Peppermint oil
- 2 drops of Neroli oil
- 2 drops of Frankincense oil
- Blank inhaler

Preparation/Application:
- Add oils to blank inhaler.
- Inhale deeply at the onset of symptoms.

Jaundice

Jaundice is a condition that refers to the yellowing of the skin and the whites of your eyes. This could mean that your liver cannot rid the body properly of bilirubin. This recipe may provide some temporary relief, but depending on the actual cause you could simply be masking a major health issue. You should always make a trip to the doctors if you are suffering from this ailment.

Ingredients:
- 2 drops Geranium oil
- 1 drop of Lemon oil
- 2 drops Rosemary oil
- 1 tbsp Extra Virgin Olive oil

Preparation/ Application:
- Dilute the essential oils with the carrier oil.
- Massage gently onto the body, on the areas most affected.

Jaw Ache

Jaw ache could be caused by the overuse of the mouth or the types of food you eat simply being tough to break down. Give your jaw a break with this easy recipe.

Ingredients:
- 3 drops of Olbas oil
- 1 drop of Juniper oil
- 2 tbsp of Avocado oil

Preparation/Application:
- Add the essential oils to two tablespoons of Avocado oil and mix well.
- Massage onto the jawline to relieve pain and loosen the jaw.

Knee Sores

Both ginger and orange oil are great at providing short term relief from pain. This recipe will reduce the pain intensity, stiffness and improve the function of your knee.

Ingredients:
- 3 drops of sweet orange oil
- 3 drops of Ginger oil
- 1 tbsp of Avocado oil

Preparation/Application:
- Mix both essential oils with the carrier oil and apply directly onto the knee sore.
- Massage well and it should take effect almost immediately once your skin soaks it up.

Leg Sores

If you experience frequent leg spasms and strain of the leg due to improper exercise or rigorous exercise, then these essential oils are for you! It's perfect for relaxing the muscles.

Ingredients:
- 3 drops of Marjoram oil
- 2 drops of Jasmine oil
- 1 tbsp of Coconut oil

Preparation/Application:
- Mix the essential oil with the coconut oil
- Apply the blend to the legs, where there is soreness.
- Massage well to relieve pain and help it absorb better.

Laundry Treatment

Sometimes when you go to clean your laundry with detergent, it doesn't seem to clean well enough. This is where essential oils come into the mix; eucalyptus provides your laundry with an added boost to freshen your clothes. Not to mention eucalyptus also diffuses the chemical irritants in detergents.

Ingredients:
- 25 drops eucalyptus oil

Preparation/Application:
-Add the essential oil to your laundry detergent and shake well.
-Eucalyptus oil has been proven to kill dust mites and is a non-allergen.

Migraine

Rosemary triggers stimulation to the scalp and brain, the musky smell and essence provides instantaneous relief to a prickling migraine.

Ingredients:
- 3 drops of Peppermint oil
- 3 drops of Rosemary oil

Preparation/Application:
- Add the essential oils to a blank inhaler.
- Inhale deeply as required.

Make-up Reaction

Essential oils are always there in times of crisis. You won't need to wait hours for the reaction to clear as essential oils get to work instantly.

Ingredients:
-3 drops Rose oil
-1 drop Orange oil
-2 drops Bergamot oil
- 1 tbsp Coconut oil

Preparation/ Application:
- Mix the essential oils with the coconut oil.
- Massage gently into the affected areas on your face.
- Be sure not to get any in your eyes.

Metabolism

Simple changes to your lifestyle can speed up weight loss and increase your metabolism rate. Take this recipe for example; with a holistic approach that creates zero side effects, not only does this method increase metabolism but it also creates a healthy self-love image.

Ingredients:
- 1 drop Lemon oil
- 1 drop Peppermint oil
- 1 drop Grapefruit oil
- 1 drop Ginger oil

Preparation/Application:
- Add these essential oils to one of the first drinks you consume each day.
- Also, add it to the final drink you have before going to sleep.

Nasal Congestion

Whenever you get hit with a cold or a blocked nose, everyone knows the go to secret is vitamin C! What better way to compliment that than by adding in the powerful healing properties of essential oils with this handy recipe.

Ingredients:
- 3 drops of Sweet Orange oil
- 2 drops of Lemon oil

Preparation/Application:
- Add the essential oils to a blank inhaler and inhale several times.
OR

- Add the essential oils into a water steamer and place your face over it. Cover with a towel and breathe in and out for several minutes.

Nail Growth

Enhance the health and length of your nails with the use of these essential oils. If you suffer from brittle nails this will also bring moisture back into them.

Ingredients:
- 1 drop of Lavender oil
- 1 drop of Rose oil
- 1 tbsp of Coconut oil

Preparation/ Application:
- Mix all the ingredients together and apply to bare nails daily.

Nausea

When overcome with a bout of nausea, all we can think of is how to make ourselves feel better. Luckily, there are some essential oils which applied on their own can provide great relief from feeling queasy. These can be administered with an inhaler which can be great to carry around with you if you are experiencing persistent nausea.

Ingredients:
- 3 drops of Peppermint oil
Or
- 3 drops of Ginger oil
Or
- 3 drops of Spearmint oil
Or
- 3 drops of Tarragon oil
- Blank inhaler

Preparation/Application:
- Add the essential oil of choice to a blank inhaler.
- Inhale deeply as required.

Neck Strain

Stress, sitting at a computer for too long or sleeping incorrectly are all major causes of neck strain. Not treating this could lead to serious consequences on the road (not being able to turn your head to check a blind spot.) Fortunately, essential oils provide a significant relief.

Ingredients:
- 1 drop of Rosemary oil
- 3 drops of Lavender oil
- 1 tbsp of carrier oil, I recommend Avocado oil.

Preparation/Application:
- Mix the essential oils with or without a carrier oil
- Massage well into the strained neck.

Odor

Whether odor in the house or body odor both are very unpleasant and can be easily kept at bay, with these simple options.

Ingredients:
- 5 drops of Roman Chamomile oil
Or
- 5 drops of Peppermint oil
Or
- 5 drops of Lemon oil
Or
- 5 drops of Jasmine oil

Preparation/ Application:
- Diffuse the essential oils in the room to improve breathing and provide a nice scent to the room.

Overeating

Essential oils have the ability to suppress cravings and nip the root causes of overeating in the bud, like; stress, anxiety, depression and insecurity. Adding a few drops of these essential oils to your water before eating will help manage your eating levels.

Ingredients:
- 2 drops of Grapefruit oil
Or
- 2 drops of Peppermint oil
Or
- 2 drops of Sandalwood oil
Or
- 2 drops of Bergamot oil

Preparation/Application:
Add 1-2 drops to a glass of water before meals.

Pet Dander

Don't suffer around animals. Diffuse essential oils in the room that you come into contact with the pets and the essential oils will keep your allergies under control.

Ingredients:
- 1 drop Thyme oil
- 2 drops Ginger oil
- 3 drops Peppermint oil

Preparation/ Application:
- Diffuse the essential oils in the room, for a lasting effect on your allergies.

Pollen Allergy

You know it's that time when you feel your allergies coming on again. But don't fret as essential oils are here to prevent your allergies from spoiling your relaxation period.

Ingredients:
- 2 drops of Peppermint essential oil
- 2 drops of Rosemary essential oil
- 1 drop of Tangerine essential oil

Preparation/ Application:
- Mix the essential oils with a tablespoon of a carrier oil of your choice.
- Store the liquid in a small tub and put it in a cool place.
- Put on a clean tissue and inhale, whenever needed.
- You could also use an inhaler for this blend.

Renal Function

Renal is just another word for kidneys. It's important to keep your kidneys healthy and busy because this is where your body filters the waste in your system. Essential oils gives the renal area the nutrients to keep them working properly.

Ingredients:
- 2 drops Ledum oil
- 1 drops Carrot Seed oil
- 1 drops Celery Seed oil
- 1 tbsp coconut oil

Preparation/ Application:
- Mix the essential oils well with the carrier oil
- Massage gently to your abdominal area, focusing on the sides where your kidneys are located.

Respiratory Function

When exposed to harmful pollutants in everyday life, it's important to give your lungs a helping hand by protecting them with essential oils. Eucalyptus contains menthol which helps clear the airway. Myrtle has been researched for its benefits in helping glandular imbalances as well.

Ingredients:
- 1 drop of Ravensara oil
- 2 drops Eucalyptus oil
- 1 drop of Pine oil
- 1 drops Myrtle oil
- 1 drops Cypress oil
- 1 tbsp Sunflower oil

Preparation/ Application:
- Mix the essential oils well with the carrier oil.
- Gently massage the blend into your chest.

Scar Remedy

Use this essential oil recipe to help reduce the appearance of scars. It will aid the skin in its long term healing process.

Ingredients:
- 3 drops Helichrysum oil
- 1 drops Myrrh oil
- 2 drops Sandalwood oil
- 1 tbsp Jojoba oil

Preparation/ Application:
- Mix well with jojoba oil and apply to scar area. Other carrier oils can be used if preferred. Scars will fade over time if applied consistently.

Skin Rash

Skin rashes are caused by viruses, bacteria, insects, heat and create itchy, irritable skin and redness, if left untreated. Essential oils possess helpful properties that'll help soothe the area and combat the issue quickly.

Ingredients:
- 3 drops of Tea Tree oil
- 3 drops of Lavender oil

Preparation/Application:
- Apply the mixture of essential oils to the skin rash.
- Massage well into the skin to relieve pain and speed up the healing process.

Sore throat

The following sore throat gargle combines the strong anti-inflammatory properties of lavender, the anti-microbial properties of eucalyptus, and the antibacterial, antiviral, and numbing properties of tea tree. *This mixture should not be swallowed, but spat out after gargling!*

Ingredients:
- 2 drops of Tea Tree oil
- 3 drops of Lavender oil
- 2 drops of Eucalyptus oil
- Glass of warm water

Preparation/Applications:
- Add oils to glass of water to create gargling solution. Stir thoroughly.
- Rinse and gargle solution by the mouthful until finished.
- Repeat every 2-3 hours, as required.

Shoulder Pain

Shoulder pain is caused by not getting enough muscle movement into the shoulder, stiffness and bad posture. Essential oils can help loosen the muscle and relieve achiness.

Ingredients:
- 1 drop of German Chamomile oil
- 3 drops of Sandalwood oil
- 1 tbsp of Avocado or Coconut oil

Preparation/Application:
- Apply the essential oils to one tablespoon of the carrier oil.
- Massage deeply into the shoulder, several times a day.

Skin Inflammation

Skin inflammation is caused when the skin is broken or damaged. Essential oils can help repair the skin tissue to make it heal fully, the natural way, without exposing your skin to chemicals.

Ingredients:
- 3 drops of Frankincense oil
- 2 drops of Rosewood oil
- 1 tbsp Coconut oil

Preparation/Application:
-Mix the essential oils thoroughly with the carrier oil.
- Apply the blend to your inflamed skin.
- Dab onto the skin with cotton wool or pad as many times as required.

Stress

Stress is caused by a number of environmental factors that can affect your mood, concentration and others around you. It is also very unhealthy to be on edge all of the time. This essential oils recipe is sure to help you relieve stress, taking advantage of the sedative properties.

Ingredients:
- 3 drops of Frankincense oil
- 2 drops of Roman Chamomile oil

Preparation/ Application:
- Mix the ingredients well together and inhale from a blank inhaler whenever you feel the need to de-stress.

Sores

Sores are caused by poor nutrition, a weak immune system and many other health issues. When left untreated they can be exceptionally painful. Essential oils can help you deal with the healing process to relieve the pain and speed up recovery.

Ingredients:
- 3 drops of Rosewood oil
- 3 drops of Lavender oil
- 1 tbsp of Coconut oil

Preparation/Application:
- Mix the essential oils well with the carrier oil
- Gently massage the blend onto your sores.
- You can do this daily until they heal.

Stomach Ache

Stomach ache is related to issues in the digestive system and poor diet as well as quite a few other things. Essential oils are really effective at getting rid of pain and discomfort. Try the recipe below to find out the benefits.

Ingredients:
- 3 drops of Tea Tree oil
- 2 drops of Lemongrass oil
- 1 tbsp of Watermelon Seed oil

Preparation/Application:
- Mix the essential oils well with the carrier oil into a small bowl.
- Massage the blend into your stomach area.

Stained Clothing

Get rid of tough stains with this essential oils recipe.

Ingredients:
- 2 drops of Lemongrass oil

Preparation/Application:
- Add the essential oil on a stain. Rub it into the fabric and allow it to sit on the stain for a few minutes before placing it inside a washing machine.

Sunburn

Sunburn is damaged skin caused by UV rays from the sun. Peppermint and eucalyptus essential oils are good for providing pain relief due to the cooling effect they give the sensitive area.

Ingredients:
- 1 drop of Peppermint oil
- 1 drop of Eucalyptus oil
- 1 tbsp of Avocado oil

Preparation/Application:
- Mix the essential oils with the carrier oil.
- Add the oils to the area of damaged skin.
- Apply daily until the sunburn is relieved and healed.

Swollen Ankles

Swollen ankles are caused when the feet have been under immense pressure from standing and walking, especially with painful shoes that are too small or very high. Essential oils are known to be pain relieving and soothing to affected areas.

Ingredients:
- 3 drops of Peppermint oil
- 3 drops of Ginger oil
- 1 tbsp of Avocado oil

Preparation/Application:
- Mix the essential oils with a tablespoon of avocado oil.
- Massage it well into the swollen ankles for instant soothing.

Sweating

Sweating can be caused by a number of factors such as heat, stress and tension. Tea tree oil is a well-known astringent and deodorant which can help fight fungal infections as well as deodorizing.

Ingredients:
- 2 drops of Tea tree oil

Preparation/Application:
- Apply onto the sweat glands with a cotton pad.
- You can apply this throughout the day as many times as needed.

Swollen Lymph Nodes

The body's lymphatic system consists of lymph vessels and lymph nodes. If the lymph nodes become swollen they can be really uncomfortable and unpleasant. Use this recipe to relieve pain and heal the lymphatic tissue.

Ingredients:
- 3 drops of Peppermint oil
- 1 drops of Lemon oil
- 1 tbsp of Grapeseed oil

Preparation/Application:
- Mix the ingredients together.
- Massage gently into the affected areas.

Self-Acceptance

Essential oils can help give you a high sense of self-worth and acceptance. There are plenty of essential oils that can be used here but I will just highlight some of my favourites.

Ingredients:
- 5 drops of Bergamot oil
Or
-5 drops of Jasmine oil
Or
- 5 drops of Orange oil
Or
- 5 drops of Rosemary oil

Preparation/Application:
- Place the essential oil in a diffuser and diffuse into the room you will be relaxing in.
- Alternatively put the essential oil into a blank inhaler and take a few inhalations when required.

Self-Confidence

Essential oils can help give you self-confidence, this recipe is to be used through diffusion.

Ingredients:
- 3 drops spearmint oil

Preparation/Application:
Use aromatically during the day, by inhaling from the bottle or diffusing.

Sugar Cravings

Sugar cravings are caused by poor nutrition or emotional distress. Use essential oils to regulate cravings and satiety.

Ingredients:
- 2 drops Roman Chamomile oil

Preparation/Application:
- Add the drops to a glass of water and drink several times a day or inhale from the bottle as you wish.

Teeth Grinding

Teeth grinding usually happens when you aren't aware of it, like when you're asleep but you can often feel the effects the following morning. Diffuse these essential oils before bed in the room or apply onto your pillow.

Ingredients:
- 2 drops Lavender oil
- 2 drops Ginger oil
- 1 drop Marjoram oil
- 2 drops Tea Tree oil
- 1 drop Thyme oil
- 1 tbsp of Coconut oil (if applying to gums)

Preparation/ Application:
- If diffusing, simply put the oils into a diffuser and use throughout the night.
- If you are applying to your pillow, drop the oils onto the side you sleep on a couple of hour before sleeping. If you find the aroma to be too strong then just flip your pillow over.
- Finally, if applying to your gums, mix the essential oils thoroughly with your carrier oil and then gently rub into your gums to help prevent the grinding.

Thrush

Essential oils are vital for this problem as they are great a providing immediate relief and don't form a resistance to yeast or bacteria.

Ingredients:
- 1 drop Thyme oil
- 2 drops Rosewood oil
- 1 drop Roman Chamomile oil
- 1 tbsp Vegetable oil

Preparation/ Application:
- Dilute with the carrier oil and apply to the roof of your mouth.

Tonsillitis

Tonsillitis is caused by viral and bacterial infections. Essential oils are antibacterial which enable them to combat the infection and also provide pain relief at the same time.

Ingredients:
- 2 drops Ginger oil
- 1 drop Lavender l oil
- 1 drop Lemon oil
- 2 drops Tea Tree oil
- 1 drop Roman Chamomile oil
- 1 tbsp Coconut oil

Preparation/ Application:
- Mix the essential oils well with the coconut oil.
- Apply the blend to the outside of your throat via a very gentle massage.

Uplifting

Lift your mood with the use of essential oils. Chamomile is calming and is an antidepressant, mood booster.

Ingredients:
- 5 drops of Roman Chamomile oil

Preparation/Application:
- Diffuse in the room you spend a lot of time in or inhale from a bottle.

Wound treatment

All of us have experienced a nasty cut, wound or scrape at some point in our lives – be it from a misguided knife during dinner preparation, or a badly grazed knee from a fall. The following remedy is a great way to clean and disinfect open wounds, while accelerating the natural healing process.

Ingredients:
- 500 mL warm, sterile water (boiled is fine)
- 2 drops of Tea Tree oil
- 5 drops of Lavender oil

Preparation/Application:
- Dilute the Tea Tree and Lavender oils in the water.
- Wash the wound generously with the solution.
- Cover wound with a gauze bandage.
- Repeat treatment twice daily, allowing time for the wound to breathe before reapplying bandage.

Window Cleaner

Use this powerful method to naturally clean your windows, leaving them shiny and polished.

Ingredients:
- 10 drops of Lemon oil
- 1 cup of White Vinegar
- Appropriate amount of Water

Preparation/Application:
- Add water and 1 cup of distilled white vinegar inside a spray bottle until it is ¾ full. Shake it well to combine both ingredients.
- Add the lemon oil to it and shake once more. Spray on the windows that need cleaning and wipe off using a paper towel.

Weight Loss

Manage your weight with the use of essential oils. They are great for lowering appetite and supressing cravings.

Ingredients:
- 2 drops Lemongrass oil

Preparation/Application:
- Add the drops of lemongrass to a glass of water in the morning and also to a glass of water in the evening.

Yeast Infection

Yeast infections can be very irritating if you leave it for too long. Essential oils are antibacterial and will help get rid of the infection.

Ingredients:
- 2 drops Lavender oil
- 3 drops Oregano oil

Preparation/ Application:
- Ingest the essential oils twice a day for up to 2 weeks until the infection goes.

The above remedies are a brief introduction into the potential therapeutic applications of essential oils. I encourage you to seek out other recipes and even experiment to create your own, especially now that you know so much more about the world of essential oils!

Essential Oils Recipes For Your Pets

Using essential oils on your pets can be a great way to naturally improve their health. They are also brilliant at masking or removing the distinct smells that pets can often leave around the house.

It is absolutely essential that you do some research on using essential oils on your pet before applying them. Cats will have an awful reaction to many essential oils and dogs whilst not as limited can still have fatal reactions to certain essential oils.

To help you make correct decisions when it comes to using essential oils and aromatherapy on your pet I have created a couple of books. These books are focused on safety.

The first, *Essential Oils For Dogs*, is available now on amazon. To find it, simply click this link or type this address into your web browser:

http://www.amazon.com/dp/B00XSDE6N8

A follow up, *Essential Oils For Cats*, will be available soon. If you sign up to my mailing list at the end of the book you will able to get it for a discounted price when it is released!

NEVER use an essential oil on your pet without doing thorough research prior. The side effects of inappropriate essential oil use on an animal can result in death.

Arthritis

Animal arthritis is caused by pain and inflammation in the joints. Treat the pain with essential oils. It will instantly relieve joint pain and discomfort.

Ingredients:
- 15 ml. of Jojoba oil
- 6 drops Rosemary oil
- 3 drops Lavender oil
- 4 drops Ginger oil

Preparation/ Application:
- Use this blend to massage your pet's sore joints. You can even apply some oil on the inside of their ears.

Treating Fleas

Fleas can hop onto your pet's fur from another pet or from infested dirt or grass outside. Once they find a host, fleas typically stay on or near this host. Fleas usually live on an animal's underbelly, so they can be easily transferred to your carpet or furnishings when your pet lies down. Control and repel fleas with this therapeutic oil treatment. This recipe will also relieve itchiness and irritation.

Ingredients:
- 4 drops of Citronella oil
- 6 drops Lemon oil
- 6 drops Clary Sage oil
- 10 drops of Peppermint oil
- 1tbsp of Olive oil

Preparation/ Application:

- Use this blend over your pet's neck, legs, tail, back and chest. You may even want to add a few drops to their collar.

Calming Your Hyperactive Pet

Relax and calm your pet down with essential oils. If
your dog seems hyper, or overly-excited, the problem likely stems
from a lack of stimulation. It is a very effective way of settling
them.

Ingredients:

- 6 drops Valerian oil
- 4 drops Lavender oil
- 2 drops Roman Chamomile oil
- 4 drops Sweet Marjoram oil
- 4 drops Bergamot oil
- 1 tbsp. of Jojoba oil

Preparation/ Application:

- This blend must be used topically. You can rub four drops of
this blend between your hands and then apply it on your dog's
ears, under their armpits and between the thighs.

Skin Allergies

Calm your pet's allergies and reduce irritation during the most unpleasant times.

Ingredients:
- 20 ml. of Sweet Almond oil
- 10 drops Lavender oil
- 5 drops Geranium oil
- 6 drops Chamomile oil
- 2 drops Carrot Seed oil

Preparation/ Application:
- Use this blend topically. You can rub four drops of this blend between your hands and then apply it on your pet's ears, under their armpits and between the thighs.

Rheum

If your feline's nose is running, consider inhalations of diluted eucalyptus oil.

Ingredients:
- 2 drops of Eucalyptus oil
- Hot water

Preparation/ Application:
- Dilute in a big bowl of hot water, and let your cat breathe in the steam. Be very careful, since the animal can occasionally burn itself.

Dry Paw Pads

The most common cause of cracked pads is over-licking, which creates a vicious self-induced cycle of irritation, redness and inflammation. If this incessant licking and scratching continues, it can lead to raw skin, sores, and infection. If your cat suffers from dry skin on the paw pads, which cracks and bleeds.

Ingredients:
- 1 drop of Lavender oil
- 60-70 drops of Coconut oil

Preparation/ Application:
- Mix well together and apply a little bit of this mixture on your cat's paws using a cotton pad.
- Also, consider putting special socks on your cat paws for a while to let the oil to be absorbed and take effect without the risk of your cat licking it. You can also use just coconut oil for this purpose.

Against Ticks

Repel ticks from your pet. They are very harmful and cause many diseases.

Ingredients:
- 1 drop of Lavender oil
- 50-60 drops of Olive oil.

Preparation/ Application:
- Put a few drops of the solution on the tick, let it sit for a while and then extract the tick and wipe away the excess oil.

Ear Infections

Scratching and rubbing at the ear and head shaking are common signs that your pet has an ear infection. You may also notice an abnormal odor from the ear or see redness or swelling. Most ear infections in adults are caused by bacteria and yeast, though ear mites. If your pet is suffering from an internal ear infection, try this recipe. Essential oils carry many antibacterial properties.

Ingredients:
- 1 drop of peppermint oil
- 70-80 drops of olive or coconut oil

Preparation/ Application:
- Mix well and apply a little bit of solution on the fur around your cat's ear. Peppermint oil has anti-bacterial properties, which will help fight the diseases.

Cleaning the Litter Box

To get rid of smell in the clean litter box use this effective method.

Ingredients:
- 1 cup of white vinegar
- 2 drops of lavender oil

Preparation/ Application:
- Use vinegar while cleaning it and spray with the solution with lavender oil diluted in a bottle of water. Rinse it with water.

Mosquito Repellent

In hotter months, get mosquitoes away from your pet when they're outside with this essential oils recipe.

Ingredients:
- 30 drops of Citronella oil
- 12 drops of Lemongrass oil
- 12 drops of Rose Geranium oil
- 12 drops of Myrrh oil
- 10 ounces of Aloe Vera juice

Preparation/ Application:
- Spray this over your pet's coat, carefully avoiding the eye area

Motion Sickness

If you are planning to travel, apply essential oils to your pet to avoid motion sickness.

Ingredients:
- 20 ml. of Jojoba oil
- 8 drops of Ginger oil
- 12 drops of Peppermint oil

Preparation/ Application:
- Apply this blend on your pet's ears, coat, thighs and armpits.
- Apply before the trip.

Sinus Infection

Caused by bacterial infections. Clear your pet's sinuses with this simple yet effective method with essential oils. They are antibacterial and are particularly useful for this issue.

Ingredients:
- 20 ml. of Sweet Almond oil
- 10 drops of Eucalyptus oil
- 6 drops of Myrrh oil
- 8 drops of Ravensare oil

Preparation/ Application:
- You can massage this blend into the fur of your pet's neck and chest. You can also add this blend into a diffuser and let your dog experience it for around ten minutes four times a day.

Pet Shampoo

Give your pet natural fur care with this recipe to avoid irritation if they're not   already experiencing it.

Ingredients:
- 10 drops Geranium oil
- 5 drops Ylang Ylang oil
- 8 drops Petitgrain oil
- 8 drops Rose oil

Preparation/ Application:
- The above blend must be added to eight ounces of all natural shampoo.

Fresh Breath

Germs and bacteria cause bad breath. Give your pet fresh breath with this essential oils recipe. It is antibacterial and extremely helpful to this cause

Ingredients:
- 20 ml. Sweet Almond oil
- 6 drops Peppermint oil
- 8 drops Coriander Seed oil
- 10 drops of Cardamom oil

Preparation/ Application:
-Mix the essential oils with the carrier oil in a small glass bottle.
- Use a dropper to give three drops to your pet every day. You will fall in love with the manner in which your pet drools over this blend.

Soothe Teething Pain

Soothe painful gums when they're teething. This blend has anti-inflammatory and anti-microbial properties.

Ingredients:
- 20 ml. Sweet Almond oil
- 6 drops Myrrh oil
- 4 drops Roman Chamomile oil
- 20 drops Clove Bud Infusion oil

Preparation/ Application:
- You could add several drops of this blend onto a frozen soft toy, so that they can chew and relieve themselves, as they play with the toy.

For Fear

If your pet is feeling scared, fearful or tense, this recipe is sure to put them at ease.

Ingredients:
- 20 ml. Sweet Almond oil
- 1 drop Neroli oil
- 2 drop Sweet Basil oil
- 8 drops Petitgrain oil
- 2 drops Ylang Ylang oil
- 6 drops Bergamot oil

Preparation/ Application:
- Carefully blend the essential oil with the carrier oil.
- Massage a small amount onto your pet's chest.
- This is a great recipe to use if your pet suffers from separation anxiety.

Treat Congestion

Congestion is commonly caused by a respiratory tract infection. Treat it with this essential oils recipe.

Ingredients:
- 15 ml. Sweet Almond Base oil
- 5 drops Eucalyptus oil
- 5 drops Myrrh oil
- 5 drops Ravensare oil

Preparation/ Application:
- The above mentioned blend must be used in a nebulizing diffuser, five to ten minutes at a time for at least four times in a day.

Strengthen the Immune System of Your Pet

The immune system is the first line of defense and should be strong at all times, so that your pet is not prone to infections and diseases. If they're feeling weak, apply this essential oils recipe to them.

Ingredients:
- 15 ml. Sweet Almond oil
- 2 drops Ravensare oil
- 2 drops Thyme oil
- 2 drops Coriander seed oil
- 2 drops Niaouli oil
- 2 drops Eucalyptus oil
- 2 drops Bay Laurel essential oil

Preparation/ Application:
-Mix the essential oil with the carrier oil.
- Massage gently onto the pets chest and back.

Coat Care

Give your pet soft and smooth fur. This recipe will also protect their coat and keep it cleaner for longer, while also making it smell nice.

Ingredients:
- 2 drops Grapefruit Seed oil
- 4 drops of Rosemary oil

Preparation/ Application:
- Use this blend in your dog's all natural shampoo to witness a soft and smooth fur.

Increasing Appetite

It can be very distressing when your dog won't eat. There are a variety of reasons for loss of appetite in dogs. Maybe you've bought a different variety of food that they'd normally eat. Because loss of appetite in pets can indicate illness, it is important to give them this recipe so that can adjust before they put them back onto their normal diet plan.

Give your pet a helping hand with this essential oils remedy. If they are not eating their regular meals.

Ingredients:
- 2 drops of Ginger oil
- 4 drops of Lemon oil
- 2 drops of Cardamom oil
- 1 drop of Spearmint oil

Preparation/ Application:
- Use this blend over your pet's paws and notice them drool over it. Using it twice a day can help in yielding results in a week's time.

Eyesight

Your canine can adapt to not being able to see, as they will rely on their other senses. However, if possible, the problem should be detected and treated. Improve your pet's vision with this essential oils recipe.

Ingredients:
- 15 ml. of Sweet Almond oil
- 2 drops Rosemary oil
- 2 drops Cypress oil
- 4 drops Frankincense oil

Preparation/ Application:
- This is an amazing blend to facilitate improvement of eyesight in your elderly pet.
- Mix the essential oils well with the carrier oil.
- Massage gently onto the chest and back of your pet.

Let me finally highlight once more that you should NEVER use an essential oil on your pet without doing thorough research prior. The side effects of inappropriate essential oil use on an animal can result in death.

Conclusion

Thank you again for choosing the read this book!

I hope this book was able to provide you with an interesting introduction into the world of aromatherapy, and to encourage you to explore the therapeutic application of essential oils further.

With everything you have hopefully learned from this guide, the next step is to put the above information to practical use, and to try and build your knowledge of essential oils even further. Be sure to keep an eye out for our more detailed guides on aromatherapy and other natural health remedies, targeted at more experienced users.

Take a few months now to build your collection of oils, gain some experience and begin to understand how the individual oils effect you. Once you feel confident with the common essential oils, begin to branch out and utilize the less common but equally effective essential oils out there.

While essential oils are generally thought of as a safer option to potentially harmful and toxic prescriptions, safety is still an issue. These powerful oils are actually concentrated, which can lead to serious damage to your health if not used properly and responsibly. To show you just how concentrated these oils are; it takes a whopping 256 pounds of peppermint leaves to get a mere 1 pound of its essential oil. Now that is some powerfully concentrated oil! Because of the high level of concentration, you really only need to use a small amount of the oil. Furthermore, almost all essential oils should be diluted if it will come in contact with the skin.

Some essential oils – such as orange, lemon, lime, grapefruit and bergamot – cause the skin to become more sensitive to sunlight (UV light). This condition is known as photosensitivity and can cause blistering and discoloration to the skin. It can also leave your skin more susceptible to burning from the sun. In order to avoid photosensitivity, never apply essential oils known to cause this problem within a 12 hour period when your skin will become exposed to sunlight.

Most experts would suggest that you avoid using essential oils on babies and children unless you get the okay from a trusted doctor. If you do use essential oils on your little ones, always exercise extreme caution and dilute the oils more so than you would for an adult. The skin of babies and children are more sensitive than that of an adult, and essential oils that are safe can actually damage their skin. However, there are a few essential oils that experts agree are safe, if used properly, for use on babies and children. These oils include chamomile, lavender, frankincense, lemon and orange. With that said, you should never use peppermint, eucalyptus, wintergreen or rosemary essential oil on babies and children.

Essential oils should be avoided when pregnant or nursing. This is because essential oils have shown to have an effect on hormones, gut bacteria and various other important body aspects that may be harmful or dangerous to the baby in the womb. If, however, you decide to go ahead and use essential oils during this time, you must always proceed with extreme caution. And never use any essential oils without first getting the okay from your doctor.

With that said, there are several oils that experts agree are not safe for use at any time during pregnancy, and should never be used. Rosemary, sage, cinnamon, basil, angelica, black pepper, aniseed, clary sage, chamomile, camphor, clove, fennel, ginger, horseradish, mustard, jasmine, juniper, nutmeg, mugwort, peppermint, marjoram, myrrh, thyme and wintergreen are among the essential oils that pregnant women should avoid at all cost.

A good general rule of thumb is to talk to your doctor or midwife about essential oils before using if pregnant or nursing. They will be able to give you their expert opinion on whether or not an essential oil should be used.

Keep in mind that not every brand of essential oil is created equal and you should always aim to use high quality oils from a reputable merchant. Furthermore, you should only use therapeutic grade or organic 100-percent pure essential oils. These oils are created using non-chemical process – such as steam distillation – and are considered safe to use both internally and externally.

Finally, if you enjoyed this book, then I'd like to ask you for a favor, would you be kind enough to leave a review for this book on Amazon? It'd be greatly appreciated!

Thank you and good luck!

2 FREE eBooks for you!

Guys, thanks so much for reading my book. I truly hope it served as a great introduction to the essential oils and aromatherapy. As a token of appreciation I have prepared two free ebooks for you. Here is a bit of information about them!

The 10 Most Important Essential Oils

In this book we delve deep into the uses and applications of the ten essential oils that I consider to be the most 'essential'. It is the natural progression from this beginner's guide that you have just read. For each oil I explain the key health benefits, teach you the therapeutic applications and provide specific safety precaution. I include one of my most useful remedies for each of the oils as well. So you will receive a deep knowledge of ten essential oils and ten brilliant remedies for free! It is a 10k word eBook, the same length as this one!

When you receive this ebook you will also receive a couple of emails from me a week containing even more information about the essential oils! I will endeavor to give you at least 5 recipes or remedies per week and also provide you with some great information on the lesser known essential oils.

Type this link into a web browser: http://bit.ly/1EuHgyn

The Ultimate Guide To Vitamins

This is another wonderful 10k word ebook that has been made available to you through my publisher, Valerian Press. As a health conscious person you should be well aware of the uses and health benefits of each of the vitamins that should make up our diet. This book gives you an easy to understand, scientific explanation of the vitamin followed by the recommended daily dosage. It then highlights all the important health benefits of each vitamin. A list of the best sources of each vitamin is provided and you are also given some actionable next steps for each vitamin to make sure you are utilizing the information!

As well as receiving the free ebooks you will also be sent a weekly stream of free ebooks, again from my publishing company

Valerian Press. You can expect to receive at least a new, free ebook each and every week. Sometimes you might receive a massive 10 free books in a week!

Type this link into a web browser: http://bit.ly/1EuHgyn

Check Out My Other Essential Oils Books!

Essential Oil Massage Techniques

Essential Oils For Allergies

Essential Oils For Dogs

Lavender Essential Oil

To find these books simply search for "Amy Joyson" in the Kindle Store!

About The Author

Hey there! I'm Amy Joyson, a lifelong student of holistic and alternative medicine. My journey began as far back as I can remember, my mother, a practicing aromatherapist, taught me value of natural remedies as a youngster. I don't think I could imagine a life without the essential oils if I tried, they are just so important to me. I am passionate about sharing their value with as many people as possible, which led me to writing my books. If you have read any of my books I truly hope they have added value to your life and I thank you with all my heart for trusting in me.

Outside of being an author, I work as a personal trainer. Employing my deep knowledge of alternative treatments has enabled me to provide outstanding results for all of my clients!

In my spare time you will often find me lounging in my hammock reading the latest aromatherapy magazine or romantic fiction novel. I have a soft spot for true romance! I aim to meditate at least once a day, and practice yoga 5 times a week. My biggest hobby however is exploring the beautiful world that we live in. Next on my hit list is Iceland, there is something seriously alluring about that island.

You can find me here on Facebook:

https://www.facebook.com/pages/Amy-Joyson/435155886642915

You can find me here on Twitter:

https://twitter.com/Amy_Joyson

Valerian Press

At Valerian Press we have three key beliefs.

Providing outstanding value: We believe in enriching all of our customers' lives, doing everything we can to ensure the best experience.

Championing new talent: We believe in showcasing the worlds emerging talent by giving them the platform to grow.

Simplicity and efficiency: We understand how valuable your time is. Our products are stream-lined and consist only of what you want. You will find no fluff with us.

We hope you have enjoyed reading Amy's guide to Lavender Essential Oil

We would love to offer you a regular supply of our free and discounted books. We cover a huge range of non-fiction genres; diet and cookbooks, health and fitness, alternative and holistic medicine, spirituality and plenty more.

All you need to do is simply type this link into your web browser: http://bit.ly/18hmup4

Preview Of My Follow Up Book "Essential Oil Massage Techniques For Beginners"

Chapter 4 –Stress relief

Stress is one of the most debilitating and prolific health risks in society today. There is a proven and commonly accepted link between stress and poor health, yet many of us accept stress as just a part of our everyday lives. Our fast paced, high stakes, 'always on' world means that there is little (if any!) down time in many people's day-to-day schedules. Sadly, it is not an uncommon experience to feel as though you are holding on by your fingernails as life whips around you, while telling yourself that the one or two weeks of holiday planned in the distant future will be enough to keep you sane for another year. Fortunately, even though we may not be able to do a lot to change the things causing stress in our lives, we can take some steps to minimize the natural stress response of our bodies. There is perhaps no better way to calm one's nerves and elevated stress levels, than with a long, relaxing massage. As mentioned above, human touch can be highly effective in making us feel calm, a fact which is made possible through the hormonal chemistry of the human body. Prolonged touch between two people has been shown stimulate the release of the bonding chemical, oxytocin. This hormone is released in high doses through events in which human contact typically occurs, including hugging, kissing, sex and even light touch between two people. Most interestingly, at least when it comes to controlling our stress levels, oxytocin has been shown to have a *suppressant* effect on the body's stress hormone, cortisol. So that means that the more we expose ourselves to physical interactions with other people, the less cortisol induced stress we are likely to feel. When the stress relieving properties of certain essential oils are added into the mix, massage can provide a much needed reprieve for even the most cortisol stricken individuals. We'll now take a look at some of the most effective oils, blends and treatments for stress relief through the combination of aromatherapy and massage.

One of the best essential oils for inducing feelings of calm is lavender. Lavender is great for a whole range of therapeutic conditions – in fact, it is an absolutely *essential* essential oil. There are lots of essential oils that have loads of excellent and varied remedial properties, however, lavender is really queen when it comes to the world of aromatherapy. It is wonderfully versatile and can be applied for a range of purposes: from disinfecting wounds, to burns treatment, to pain relief. It is also one of the very few essential oils that can safely be applied to the skin 'neat' or undiluted. In summary, if you had to choose a 'desert island' essential oil, lavender should naturally be the go to option! Not least among the valued properties of lavender, is its ability to be utilized as an effective treatment for stress relief. Thanks to the versatility of lavender, we'll talk more about this special oil later on, but for now it is important to remember – *lavender is great for inducing a sense of calm.* Clary sage is another essential oil that has a particularly good effect in calming a patient's nerves. Derived from the steam distilled buds and leaves of the Clary Sage plant (*Salvea Sclarea),* this essential oil exhibits many parallel and complementary properties to lavender, especially when it comes to inducing a calmative effect. This remarkable herb has long been valued in its own right for its many and varied medicinal qualities, including its effect as an antidepressant, sedative and nervine agent. Care should be taken when using clary sage in combination with alcohol, as the herb can intensify the effects of this drug. Finally, geranium oil has been shown to be a highly effective emotional 'balancing' agent, which can greatly assist those suffering from anxiety or depression.

With the above calm inducing essential oils in mind, we'll now take a look at how to combine these into a great massage blend for stress relief. When making a blend for stress relief, it is perfectly acceptable to use a fairly neutral carrier oil, such as grapeseed as the primary constituent. This is because the essential oils are really doing the lion's share of the work here, and work in two distinct ways to create a feeling of calm. First, the scent of the essential oils works through the body's olfactory system to stimulate the limbic system, and helps to regulate impulses from the central nervous system that lead to an overactive adrenal response. For this reason, a carrier oil with a relatively neutral scent should be used here. The volatile compounds of the active essential oils also work by entering the body through the bloodstream; from here, they circulate throughout the body where they can relax muscles and also influence cortisol and adrenaline levels in the body by limiting overactive stress hormone production. As such, opting for a carrier oil with a moderately good rate of absorption (such as grapeseed or apricot kernel oils) is recommended.

With this in mind, the following treatment makes for a good remedy when treating stress in a patient: 3 drops of clary sage oil; 3 drops of lavender oil; 3 drops of geranium oil; 10mL grapeseed oil. All ingredients should be combined in a dark glass jar and shaken to combine. When applying via massage, the applicant should take a small amount of the blend (about the size of a dime) and rub together in their palms to warm before applying to the patient. Focus the massage on the back and shoulders, which can carry a lot of tension in a person experiencing high levels of stress. If you have more time, a full body massage can provide great benefits to a patient suffering from stress. Apply the same technique to the legs, arms, back, neck, shoulders, feet, hands and head. A comprehensive massage such as this (which can take around 45 minutes to an hour) can ensure the complete relaxation of the recipient as they become fully immersed in the experience. Good results can also be achieved using what is known as the *raindrop technique* which will be discussed further in the later chapter on meditation.

Type this link into your web browser:

http://amzn.to/1C5NDCf

Made in the USA
San Bernardino, CA
05 January 2016